What's a Woman to Do?

Practical Answers to Women's Healthcare Questions in the 21st Century

Dr. Steven M. Willis

PublishAmerica
Baltimore

First printing

ISBN: 1-4137-4901-1
PUBLISHED BY PUBLISHAMERICA, LLLP
www.publishamerica.com
Baltimore

Printed in the United States of America

To my children: Heather, Grant, Glenn, and Kathleen: who have learned that knowledge is a key to opening the vast unknown.

The mind of the prudent acquires knowledge,
And the ear of the wise seeks knowledge...
Proverbs 18:15 (NAS)

Acknowledgments

I wish to thank the following individuals for their assistance in this project: my wife and best friend, Genie, for her love, encouragement, (and hot flashes) to initially undertake this project; Ginny Anthony for her editorial and artistic assistance; Camille Patton for cool computer tricks; longtime friend and business partner Ronald Hoffman, DC; nurse practitioner Julie Holt, ARNP, family practice doctors Patricia Hogan, MD & Laura Rosner, MD, Nancy Long, Regional VP Arbonne International, and Linda Miles, Ph.D. for assistance and information from their respective fields; Cathy Corredor for years of transcription assistance, and finally my office staff Darlene McRae and Stephanie Branch for putting up with all the interruptions in a normal day of patient care.

A Word of Caution

The information contained on the CD and in the text is intended for informational and educational purposes. While most of the recommendations are applicable to the general population, they are not intended to take the place of medical evaluation and treatment. The success of a portion of the program is based on proper laboratory and clinical monitoring. You are encouraged to discuss any changes in your health status with your physician.

Table of Contents

Part Five—Prescription Estrogen (and other hormones)

Part Six—Nutrition

Part Seven—Putting It All Together

Foreword

In February of 2000, I almost died of complications from pneumonia. I was 52. After a year, I still felt weary and spent. I realized that I had insurance to cover *illness,* but not to cover *wellness.* I then turned to alternative healthcare practitioners—Dr. Steven Willis, chiropractor, and Dr. Min Tian. Finally, I began to feel whole and healthy. This book is the recipe that gave me back my vitality and spirit.

When Dr. Willis uses the ABCs—About Being Complete, I applaud his analysis and practicality. As my life zips along, I am a testimonial since I became ill as a result of not taking care of myself. I have learned to live in the present and not overdo. In order to restore and energize my metabolism, I follow the wellness program outlined in this book.

"Wisdom begins with wonder" (Socrates). Dr. Willis is a continuous learner, searching for the best practices in women's health. I admire him for asking questions, doing research, and promulgating practical solutions for a woman's healthy lifestyle. He is a seeker and a healer. Candice Pert. Ph.D. in her text, *Molecules of Emotion*, states it effectively in describing her goal, "I seek to inform, to educate, and inspire all manner of people, from lay to professional. I try to make available and interpret the latest and most up-to-date knowledge… information that is practical, that can change peoples lives." Dr. Willis works and writes by a like goal.

What's a Woman to Do? provides cutting-edge information about what pollutes our bodies, and how to achieve a healthy lifestyle. In this is a guide for restoration and preservation of health, where Dr. Willis uses a wonderful metaphor about a stream. As he notes, it is much easier to deal with a problem—at the beginning of the stream, rather than after the stream has become polluted and contaminated.

Based on my own personal experience and professional association with Steve, I highly recommend this book to women who are seeking answers about maintaining their weight, health, and sense of well-being. Mother Teresa once said, "Our best protection is a joyful heart." Being healthy allows us to face life's challenges with a joyful and healthy heart.

Linda D. Miles, Ph.D.
Psychotherapist and Author of *The New Marriage.*

Introduction

What's a Woman to Do?

"What's a Woman to Do?" was the title of a two-page paper I wrote in mid 2002. It was in response to numerous inquires from my female patients after the Women's Health Initiative study on hormone replacement therapy was terminated early. Additionally, I was spending time in two friends' medical offices observing their gynecology and family practices and heard the same questions posed to them. Not surprising, at that time they did not have any better answer for their patients than I had for mine.

It is said, "necessity is the mother of invention." The same can be said for frustration. In late 2001, my wife remarked how frustrating it was that she could not find one doctor who could act as a resource for the questions related to menopause, diet and nutrition, exercise, and the other issues related to "getting older." As a chiropractor, I had confined the majority of my practice to sports and spinal related healthcare. I had spent the first 15 years of my practice as a team physician for a local high school and a period with FSU's women's track. Around the same time (2001), I was feeling intellectually frustrated and accepted my wife's challenge to be that resource for my patients. Out of all of this came a lecture series on hormones, diet/nutrition and exercise/stress reduction, an instructional CD and, finally, this book.

How to Use the CD and Book

This book can be of value with or without the accompanying CD. If you do not have a copy of the CD, you may obtain one by contacting:

Steven M. Willis, D.C.
1911 Buford Blvd.
Tallahassee, FL 32308
850.878.3999

Include check or money order for $15 plus $5 S&H or call 850.878.3999t to place an MC/VISA order.
or
Go to www.chirowomenwellness.com for additional information and to preview the CD.

If you have not reviewed the CD or do not have a copy, you will start this book a little differently—from the back to the front. Finish reading this section, and then please read Part 7, "Putting It All Together." Familiarize yourself with the basics and follow the instructions to pick one item in each of the application choices. Do not be overwhelmed; start to think about healthy lifestyle changes. After completing the instructions in Part 7, return to the beginning, and read the book starting with Part 1. The remainder of the text will help your understand "why you want to change."

READ ON!

Groundwork. Preplanning. Whatever you call "it," it takes some of "it," in order to successfully get from here to there. Think about the last vacation that resulted in wonderful memories. You did a lot of research and planning. I want you to begin to think of health as a journey - a journey from where you are today to where you want your health to be sometime in the future.

Often, an individual will become so overwhelmed with the choices and decisions related to a trip that they become confused and frustrated before beginning. It is even worse when it comes to making health related decisions. Candice Pert, Ph.D., notes it is her experience that most people seeking health related answers want to have science demystified, de-jargonized, and described in terms that they can understand. I hope to make the process of decision making easier. K.I.S.S.—keep it simple stupid! That is the cry I hear from patients. The problem is the body is not simple. In theory every automobile, of the same make and model, should be the same. The plans and parts are all the same. With the body, the generalized plan and parts are the same, but the actual construction is highly variable. In treating the body, whether by physician or self, it is soon evident that what works for one individual does not necessarily work for another person. LESSON NUMBER 1 in the health journey is to realize that it will take time and that modifying the initial plan is a reality.

Dr. Barry Sears in his book, *The Omega Rx Zone*, notes that to move toward health you must macro-manage wellness, not micro-manage disease. This will be a recurring theme throughout this book. Our goal is HEALTH and WELLNESS, not just the removal of symptoms.

Another recurring theme will be the importance of "balance." Within medicine the term is homeostasis. Homeostasis is defined as the state of equilibrium (balance between opposing pressures). I present a balanced approach to the areas of stress reduction, hormone balance, exercise, and nutrition. There are no "magic bullets" to regain health. Maintaining the balance of health will require monitoring and change.

One goal is to weed through the complexity of healthcare issues and present those issues that allow you to make wise choices in the journey to health. I will try to K.I.S.S. Some may find it more information than they want to know. Remember that good decisions are made from a position of knowledge. You have the ability to understand more than you may give yourself credit for. Others, those with a science/medical background, may find the information too basic. The book addresses relevant issues, understandable to the population addressed, covering modifiable conditions that allow the individual to measure change. The information is not meant to replace clinical healthcare advice. The material provides recommendations that will improve the health status of all women.

Note the text and CD are divided into sections. The CD parallels the text and, in addition to being an easy first introduction to the material, may be used as a teaching and lecture aid. The first section covers an overview of various relevant topics including: Doctor-Patient Partnerships, the ABCs, the concept of Progressive Practical Application, and a new paradigm to challenge your approach to dealing with healthcare issues. The subsequent sections address the areas of stress reduction, environmental estrogen exposure, prescription estrogens, and nutrition. Each section contains background material and current medical findings. Because the ultimate goal of the program is to have you to make appropriate steps to health, each section ends with "Practical Application."

All the planning and web surfing will mean nothing if, for the vacation, you do not leave the house and start to the destination. Likewise, if you read this book and do not act on it, nothing in your healthcare will change. Reflecting on health as a journey, remember that every trip begins with one step. Both learning "what to do" and the "doing" are a progressive activity. Taking one step toward improved health is better than no step. Understanding and application will grow and improve as you experience health. My desire is to make sense of the components of macro-managing wellness and motivate you to make a commitment to positive life choices.

Let's Get Started

First, go through the CD one time from beginning to end. This will serve as a general introduction to the material and should take not more than 30 minutes. Do not spend much time on one area and do not try to figure out how you are going to apply the recommendations. Next, start back through; this time writing notes on the areas that will have the greatest initial impact on your health. Pay attention to the "Practical Application" sections and remember the principle of progressive application. The goal is to start with one or two recommendations and incorporate them into your lifestyle. Much like the analogy equating the learning process to a marathon, not a sprint, you should not try to "do" all the things under the application heading. Success will come when these recommendations become a natural part of your daily activities. Do too much too quickly and the only thing you will achieve is "frustration."

Having decided on the task(s) you will be working into a "lifestyle" change, set about to understand why these changes are important. Now, read the text to gain additional insight. I have tried to give enough facts and statistics to convince you of the importance of making these endeavors a lifetime commitment.

As you become comfortable with the new changes, review the recommendations and see if it is time to add to your list. You do not have to necessarily add something in each area every time. While some changes may come easily, others will be a challenge. My personal experience is that wholesale changes in the area of nutrition are the most difficult, especially if you have a family. Your spouse and/or children may not as readily accept your enthusiasm for change. Be patient...be persistent...set out to be successful in your quest and follow the recommendations.

STOP!

Except for reviewing the information on using the CD, read no further until you have worked through the CD as directed (or read Part 7 if you do not have the CD).

Come on; let's get started on the right foot!

Instructions for Running the CD in Your Computer (PC)

This program is presented in a PowerPoint format.
When viewing the presentation, you can:

· **Advance** to the next slide by striking "page down," "enter," or the space bar.
· **Return** to the previous slide by striking "page up."
· **End** the presentation by striking "Esc."

Getting Started:
If you have Power Point on your computer:

· Insert the CD into your computer's CD drive.
· If your computer automatically opens your CD drive, you will see 2 files.
Double-click on the Balancing Hormones icon.
Click on Slide Show, then View Show.

If your computer *does not* automatically open your CD drive:
    Double-click on My Computer.
    Double-click on Drive D (or your CD drive designation).
    Double-click on the Balancing Hormones icon.
    Click on Slide Show, then View Show.

If you do not have Power Point on your computer:

A Power Point Viewer program has been included on the CD but must be installed prior to viewing the slide presentation.

· Insert the CD in your computer's CD drive.
· If your computer automatically opens your CD drive, you will see 2 files.
Double-click on the Power Point Viewer icon and follow the instructions for installation. This program will remain on your computer for future use.
After installation is complete return to the CD drive interface.

Double-click on the Balancing Hormones icon.
Click on Slide Show, then View Show.

· If your computer *does not* automatically open your CD drive:
Double-click on My Computer.
Double-click on Drive D (or your CD drive designation).
Double-click on the Power Point Viewer icon and follow the instructions
for installation. This program will remain on your computer for future use.
After installation is complete return to the CD drive interface.
Double-click on the Balancing Hormones icon.
Click on Slide Show, then View Show.

Part One

The Beginning:
Knowledge is Power

In order to arrive at what you are not
You must go through the way in which you are not.
—T. S. Eliot

Women's Healthcare in the 21st Century

The last century has included major advancements in major health related issues, especially those dealing with men's healthcare. According to Harrison's *Principle's of Internal Medicine* women have been under-represented in drug trials even though women use the majority of pharmaceuticals. Studies that have included women indicate that there are significant clinical differences in the way women respond to various pharmaceuticals. In the 1992 FDA "Adverse Experience Report" it was noted that women have a higher frequency of adverse reactions to drugs than men. Today, studies and clinical trials are being separated out to note "gender based" biologic processes.

Understanding how women's health issues differ from men's is relevant when presenting a program intended to encourage lifestyle changes in the female population. Examples of misunderstanding include the difference between the sexes related to heart disease, various cancers, and the difference in medical procedures that are used to address these issues.

Confusion exists within the female population when it comes to understanding mortality. Women can expect to outlive their male counterpart by 6 years (79.1 vs. 73.1). Life expectancy is a perfect example of this perplexity. In 1900, the average life expectancy for a woman was in the mid-forties. Reasons for this average were the fact that 1 in 5 women died before the age of 5 and 1 in 40 died in childbirth. If a woman survived the childbearing years, her life expectancy was the same as today. Today's average life expectancy indicates advances in the treatment of fatal childhood illnesses and childbirth, but there has been no significant improvement in the major degenerative health issues that plague women.

There are a number of factors that affect morbidity (illness) and mortality (death). In the last 30 years in the U.S. there has been a "feminization" of poverty. One-third of families headed by women live in poverty. For African-American and Latino women the number is one-half. Statistics reveal that one-fifth of women over the age of 65 live below the poverty level. Women in lower socioeconomic levels tend to experience poorer health and higher mortality rates than women in higher income groups. Women living below the poverty level are more likely to smoke and less likely to have recommended preventative health screenings and other measures. The lack of universal insurance continues to be a major problem for women in general. Females tend to have lower paying, part-time, non-union jobs that do not typically provide health insurance benefits. Many times divorced women will lose the health benefits they had through their husband's employment.

Preventative screening and education are an important part of improving the health status of women. Recommended preventative screenings include:

1. A baseline history and physical.
2. Counseling in: diet, smoking cessation, exercise, safe sexual practices, alcohol abuse, and violence.
3. Regular screenings for breast, cervical, and colorectal cancer. Clinical breast exams (by a physician) are recommended to start at age 35. Recommendations for mammography vary, but there is consensus agreement that this should be completed annually between the ages of 50 and 59. The benefits are debatable for women between the ages of 40 and 49, but I believe a baseline exam should be completed if there are any associated risk factors for breast cancer (see risk factors below). Recent evidence reported in the *Journal of the American Medical Association* found in mammograms of women with breast augmentation, the screening missed the cancer 55% of the time. It is recommended that these women choose an imaging center that specializes in screening of augmented breasts. Because it is easier to read mammograms of older women with less dense breast tissue, annual mammograms after age 60 may not be necessary. PAP smear screening for uterine cervical cancer should be initiated at age 18 or when sexually active. After 2 to 3 normal screenings, follow-up is recommended every 3 years. For women with a 10-year negative history regular screening can be discontinued after age 65. The American Cancer Society recommends yearly fecal occult blood test after age 50. Colonoscopy is appropriate starting at age 50 or earlier if there are signs of rectal bleeding or marked changes in bowel function. Bone mineral testing (DEXA scan) is recommended starting at the time of menopause or before, if there is a strong family history of osteoporosis, the presence of major risk factors, or following the extended use of steroid medications (prednisone or cortisone).

Recommendations are per Harrison's Principle's of Internal Medicine.

Breast Cancer

Breast cancer is probably the most feared word for women when discussing health related illnesses. Women believe that breast cancer poses the greatest threat to their lives. The reality is that over one's lifetime the odds for being diagnosed with breast cancer is 1 in 8. The odds of dying from heart disease are 1 in 3. Death related to breast cancer is greatest when diagnosed in the younger woman. Leading causes of death in women (ages 25-34) are accident, HIV infection, homicide, and suicide; (ages 45-54) breast cancer, ischemic heart disease, lung cancer, and colon cancer; (ages 65-74) ischemic heart disease, lung cancer, GI cancer, and COPD. Among women of all ages ischemic heart disease is the leading cause of death by a substantial margin, with a mortality rate 5 to 6 fold higher than lung cancer or breast cancer.

The statistics related to breast cancer:

- Lifetime risk - 1 in 8
- Decreases to 1 in 13 if no first-degree relative has been diagnosed.
- Increases to 1 in 5 if two first-degree relatives have been diagnosed.

The risk of being diagnosed with breast cancer in the next 10 years:

- Age 30—1 in 249
- Age 40—1 in 67
- Age 50—1 in 36
- Age 60—1 in 29
- Age 70 - 1 in 24

The risk of getting breast cancer:

- By age 25—1 in 19,608
- By age 35—1 in 622
- By age 45—1 in 93
- By age 55—1 in 33
- By age 65—1 in 17

- By age 75—1 in 11
- By age 85—1 in 9
- Ever - 1 in 8

Source: the National Cancer Institute

When breast cancer is diagnosed in the early stages, the 5-year survival rate is greater than 95%. A report at the Society of Epidemiologic Research conference in June 2003, revealed a positive relationship between exercise and breast cancer (BCIS—breast cancer in situ). They noted that women who exercised in the prior ten years had a lower rate of BCIS. Dr. Michelle Holmes, of Brigham and Women's Hospital in Boston, has presented evidence that moderate exercise improved the survival rate from breast cancer. Women who exercised after breast cancer were noted to reduce their chance of dying by 25 to 50%. Dr. Holmes information was based on data from the Nurses Health Study.

Breast cancer risk factors include:

Established:
- Advancing age
- Early menarche—onset of periods
- Late menopause
- First-degree relative with breast cancer
- Late age at first birth
- High dose oral contraceptives
- Not breast-fed as an infant

Potential risk factors:
- Did not breast-feed own child
- Post-menopausal obesity
- Diet related factors, including low vegetable, fruit, fiber, and carotinoids intake, high fat diet. Low vitamin C and folate in diet
- High use of alcohol
- Excess caffeine intake
- Gene alteration—BRCA1, BRAC2
- Estrogen and hormone replacement therapy

Conflicting evidence:
- Pesticide exposure
- DDT exposure

- Smoking
- Ionizing radiation (x-rays)
- Benign breast disease

Suspected risk factors:
- Environmental estrogens (see Part 4).
- PCB/PBB exposure
- Electromagnetic fields (*i.e.,* high voltage transmission lines and electric blankets)
- Progestin containing oral contraceptives

Adapted from Freudenheim and Potishman, 1996.

A recent study has associated weight gain after the age of 18 with increased risk of breast cancer. The American Cancer Society (ACS) has stated that a 20-30 pound weight gain after high school increases the risk by 40%. There is a 200% increase with a 70 or more pound gain. Spencer Feigelson, senior epidemiologist at the ACS, notes that weight gain is the second leading cause of all cancers.

There are relevant findings with regard to the association of foods and breast cancer. It is clear that excess saturated fat, weight gain, and alcohol consumption increase the incidence of breast cancer. Yale University recently reported the association of obesity and the survival rate from breast cancer. They noted that obese African American females had a lower survival rate than their white counterparts. As you will read in a later section, an increase in the acidity of the tissues, as a result of diet, has been related to increased degenerative diseases and cancer. A study from Michigan State University noted an association of a decrease in consumption of cruciferous vegetables (cabbage and sauerkraut) contributed to increased breast cancer risk.

Heart Disease

Heart disease is the number one killer of women. Until recently, research into the relationship of cardiovascular disease and women was lacking and far behind that of men's. While there have been increased monies spent investigating the complexities of female heart disease, there continues to be a disconnect in public awareness of the depth of the problem. It is estimated that 40,000 women will die annually from breast cancer, while nearly 500,000 die from cardiovascular related health issues. Four hundred and forty thousand women will have a heart attack annually. A woman has a 50% chance of dying from her first heart attack as compared to 30% mortality for men. For those women who survive, 38% will have a second attack within 1 year (compared to 25% for her male counterpart). The cost to industry is higher as a result of female heart conditions, as 46% of women will be disabled (totally or temporarily) compared to 22% of men.

For too long it was accepted that women were just "small males." Current research has shown that the female structure responds differently to stress, hormones and medications, saturated fats, and environmental toxins, including smoking. On average, a woman will be diagnosed with heart disease 10 years later than a male. It has always been assumed that this was due to the protective value of estrogen on the premenopausal woman. Recent findings (see "What the Studies Say") note that there is no protection of the heart for postmenopausal women as a result of continued hormone replacement. Women who start on hormones after menopause have an increased risk of heart attack in the first year after initiation of hormones.

Physicians note a number of dissimilarities in the emergence of female heart attack compared to males. Many women do not experience the classic signs of a heart attack: shortness of breath, pain in the chest, left arm and jaw. Women may have more subtle signs, including nausea, a general feeling of illness, and symptoms too often associated with anxiety. Scientists believe that this is due to the fact that while men have marked arterial occlusion (blockage), women have spasms of the vessels that impede blood flow. It is believed that plaque material that clogs men's hearts acts differently in women. The major arterial vessels are the site for occlusion in men, while there is a more generalized (full body) deposition of plaque in women. Dr. Noel Bairey Merz, of Cedars-Sinai Medical Center in Los Angles, has noted an analogy: women distribute the "garbage" associated with arteriosclerosis in a similar fashion as weight gain. Men tend to put weight on primarily in the belly. Women on the other hand distribute the fat more evenly. This changes after menopause and as a result of Metabolic Syndrome. There are currently guidelines that calculate cardiovascular risk by evaluating body proportion including the size of the waistline in relationship to the hips. For a woman, a ratio of greater than 1:1 of waist to hip indicates increased risk for cardiovascular disease. For women, a ratio of .8 or less is considered safe. The overall waist circumference is a common measure to assess presence of excess abdominal fat. Women with a waist circumference over 35 inches are at increased risk for premature death and disability.

How to measure waist circumference: using a cloth measuring tape or string, measure the distance around the smallest area below the ribs and above the top of the pelvic bones. This should fall just above the umbilicus (belly button).

How to measure hip circumference: using a cloth measuring tape or string, measure the distance around the widest part of the buttocks.

Just like breast cancer it is important to understand the risk factors associated with an increased chance of cardiovascular involvement. These include:

·   If your father had a heart attack before age 55, or your mother before age 65.
·   Smoking
·   Diabetes
·   High blood pressure
·   Elevated cholesterol levels
·   Excess weight
·   Inactivity

In general, women tend to be overweight more than men and are affected more adversely by stress and less likely to exercise. The protective benefits to premenopausal women are totally lost as a result of smoking and diabetes. It is estimated that the majority of heart attacks in women could be prevented with a combination of lifestyle changes and proper medications when needed.

General warning signs of a heart attack as noted by the American Heart Association:

- Chest discomfort. It can feel like a squeezing or pressure in the middle of the chest. Please note that most heart attacks begin with mild discomfort, which may come and go.
- Discomfort in other areas of the upper body—arms, back, jaw, upper-stomach (epigastric pain may be confused for gastritis or reflux).
- Shortness of breath.
- Nausea, cold sweats, lightheadedness.

Warning signs of a stroke:

- Sudden weakness or numbness in the face, arms, legs, especially on one side of the body.
- Sudden confusion, or trouble speaking or understanding.
- Sudden trouble seeing.
- Sudden trouble walking, dizziness with loss of balance or coordination.
- Sudden headache without known cause.

Resource: *A Woman's Heart*, BioAging, Inc.

What can you do?

- Follow through on your intuition if you think you are having a heart attack. Women do experience more stress-related chest pain, sore chest muscles, and monthly variations of chest tenderness, and these make diagnosis more problematic.
- Be regular with thorough physical and diagnostic evaluations. The *Women's Ischemic Syndrome Evaluation* (WISE) notes that while classic treadmill tests tend to result in false-positives for many women, it may in fact be an early warning of things to come in the next 20 years. (Make lifestyle changes now!)
- Stop smoking. If you quit, your increased risk will reduce by 50% within 2 years and return to near normal within 10 years.
- Lose weight. Obesity increases the risk for diabetes.
- Lower cholesterol. Women tend to have elevated triglycerides and lower HDL (good) cholesterol. Triglycerides rise as a result of excess carbohydrate intake.
- Control blood pressure. More than ½ of women over 45 have elevated blood pressure. (120/80 is considered normal; 130/90 borderline hypertensive; 140/95 hypertensive.)
- Reduce stress. Chronic stress causes excess cortisol secretion and

increased insulin production.

· Understand the role of hormone balance. Birth control pills increase the risk in women over 35, especially if they smoke or have elevated blood pressure.

There are various tests available to monitor the development and treatment of heart disease. These include:

· Stress test: a measurement of heart function when placed under physical stress, usually accomplished with a treadmill. Cardiac status (heart electrical activity) is monitored by EKG (electrocardiogram). Additional testing may include an echocardiogram (ultrasound of the heart).

· EBCT: Electron Beam Computed Tomography. This is a variation of a CT scan that calculates the density of calcium deposits in coronary arteries. The cost is between $350 and $500 and at this time not generally covered by insurance.

· CRP: C-reactive protein. A blood test that measures a substance produced in the liver in response to injury or infection (see Your Inflammatory Status).

Additional information specific to heart health and women can be obtained from WomenHeart: the National Coalition for Women with Heart Disease at www.womenhealth.org.

Smoking

A major modifiable risk factor related to deteriorating health for women is cigarette smoking. Women that smoke have a six fold increased risk for having a heart attack than non-smoking women. Lung cancer is the leading cause of cancer death among women and kills 68,800 per year—29,000 more than breast cancer. Smoking related illness will kill 178,000 women per year. Smoking is a major cause of free radical production considered a cause of pre-cancerous and cancerous cells. There is an increased risk of cervical cancer and difficulty conceiving as a result of smoking.

One fourth of women in their thirties smoke and that makes it the highest percentage of any age group. Overall, 21% of all women smoke and are 1/3 less likely to quit than men. On average, women who smoke decrease their lifespan by 14 years (men decrease theirs by 13 years). The reasons women give for not quitting include: their concern about weight gain, emotional instability, stress reduction, used for a sense of connection (friendship), and related to their self image (most women who smoke started in their teens). A recent article from the Scientific Institute of Public Health, Brussels, Belgium, noted that young adult smokers were less likely to demonstrate other healthy nutritional habits. They tended to eat breakfast less often and consumed less fruits and vegetables. This definitively demonstrates the cumulative nature of poor health habits and the affect on total health.

Smoking is a national concern because of the effects of secondhand smoke. Credible evidence exists that relates coronary heart disease (CHD) with exposure to passive smoking. Besides the relationship of smoking to production of endocrine disruptors (EDs—see Part 4 "Environmental Estrogens") and free radicals, there is a negative affect on HDL cholesterol levels.

The issue of smoking represents the most modifiable habit that would have an immediate affect on healthcare in America. Besides the obvious personal health benefits, the cost savings to both the individual and corporate insurance carriers would be immense. With our current healthcare crisis, which includes having 1/6 of Americans uninsured and a higher percentage "underinsured," this lifestyle change represents a responsible step to slow the monetary drain of health dollars. The National Cancer Institute estimates that if people quit smoking, that measure alone would decease death from all cancers by 30%. It is estimated that the U.S. spends $64 billion annually on cancer treatment. Funds for R&D (research and development) are over $14 billion annually, including monies from the federal and state governments, and pharmaceutical companies. All together, Americans have spent nearly $200 billion since 1971 through various channels, including taxes, donations, and private R&D on cancer research.

Part Two
Health in Today's Market

The doctor said: This-and-that indicates that this-and-that is wrong with you, but if analysis of this-or-that does not confirm our diagnosis, we must suspect you of having this-or-that, then...and so on. There was only one question Ivan Ilyich wanted answered: was his condition dangerous or not? But the doctor ignored that question as irrelevant.
—Leo Tolstoy, *The Death of Ivan Ilyich*

Normal Function or a Disease Process?

How do we define health? Is it the absence of disease? When diagnosed with heart disease, diabetes, or cancer, it did not "just happen." Even today, your body is undergoing a long downward transition of changes that may eventually lead to a chronic disease state. Most of us live in the "gray" zone of sub-chronic disease where overt signs and symptoms are hidden or minimal. Our goal is to move toward wellness. In order to do this, one must macro-manage wellness, not micro-manage disease. In today's health environment of documentation, normal physiological functions have gained disease status. ICD (International Classification of Diseases) gives an identification number to concisely identify diseases and abnormal function. Under this classification, abnormal function (as well as some normal function) is equated with disease. Within the medical system "fever" is assigned a CPT code number. In reality, fever is a symptom indicating that an internal body function is taking place—the function of combating infection. Monitoring the fever can give an indication of how effective the prescribed therapy is working or not working. The goal is to aid the body in its ability to fight infection, not the elimination of the fever. Often we reach for aspirin at the first sign of fever, to reduce the symptom, instead of allowing the body to function in the way it was designed. The assumption is that once the fever is gone, the "disease" has been controlled.

Medicine is what the doctor can do for you.
Health is what you can do for yourself.

H. L. "Sam" Queen, CCN
Institute for Health Realities

The Role of Advertising in Healthcare

The statement "perception is more important than reality" is a "reality" in healthcare in America today. The perception is that taking certain medicines and eliminating symptoms leads to health. On an average night, there are 7 or more advertisements for drugs during the 30-minute evening news period. There are approximately 2500 prescriptions listed in the PDR (Physicians Desk Reference). The 10 most highly advertised drugs (Celebrex, Vioxx, numerous antidepressants, statin cholesterol lowering drugs like Zocor, Viagra, and numerous reflux meds like Nexium, "the purple pill"), sell more than the other 2490 drugs combined.

A decade ago, most drug "advertising" was done in the manner of pharmaceutical representatives (detailmen) in direct contact with physicians. Literature and samples of the newest drugs were distributed to the physician to give to patients in an effort to encourage the physician to prescribe the drug. Congress became involved when there was evidence of other incentives (gifts and trips to physicians) being used to increase sales. Limits were set on what a physician could accept without evidence of impropriety. When the rules changed, so did the manner of "advertising"—out with the doctor and direct to the consumer became the method of choice. In November of 2002, the pharmaceutical company Wyeth began a national campaign about depression on college campuses. The multibillion-dollar pharmaceutical industry knew that the college campus was a fertile and growing marketplace for sales.

An example of irresponsible usage of prescription drugs is the over reliance on antibiotics, combined with food sources exposed to xenobiotics, having contributed to the development of strains of "super bacteria." During a time when MD's are supposed to be discouraging the overuse of antibiotics, actual spending on antibiotics has increased 42%. Numerous studies have revealed that a significant number of physicians will give a patient a prescription because of the patient's expectation of what needs to be done. In fact, the number of prescriptions written for adolescents has increased (percentage wise) faster than any other age group. Spending on drugs for ADHD has risen 122% over the last 4 years according to a study by

MedcoHealth Solutions. Spending on prescription drugs to treat adolescent heartburn and GI distress has increased 660% over a five-year period. Are these drugs being prescribed to counteract the side effects of other drugs taken in adult dosages, or a result of poor nutrition (or both)? Asthma and allergies in children have more than doubled in the last decade. The removal of symptoms does not equate to health; many seemingly healthy individuals have died due to underlying/silent and progressive disease processes. We need to review our attitudes toward using pharmaceuticals for the removal of symptoms only. We may have inadvertently exacerbated the recreational drug problem in America by our casual and inappropriate attitudes to prescription medications.

Misleading, come-on advertising is not confined to the pharmaceutical industry. The food industry has been guilty of massive campaigns of "misinformation." The low-fat/no-fat craze of the last decade is a prime example. A little math will help clarify this topic (the section on nutrition will discuss this in additional detail). A gram of carbohydrate or protein is 4 calories. A gram of fat is 9 calories. When the American Heart Association went on a lipid (cholesterol) lowering campaign, "fat" mistakenly became the prime villain. Food companies produced low fat everything with the end result that Americans became fatter. Lost in the advertising blitz that low-fat foods were better for you, was the reality that while all food grams are not equal, in the end, calories are calories. The inclusion of good fat in foods is one of the factors that create satisfaction with the food eaten. Without the element of satisfaction, individuals tend to continue to eat. In reality, what was exchanged was a decrease in calories from fat, but a marked increase in total calories consumed, primarily from carbohydrates. Remember the jingle, "Bet you can't eat just one!" That was the mantra of the fat-free bag of chips and cookies. Somehow, "serving size" awareness got lost in translation.

The current craze is the *low-carb* diet. The importance in understanding this method of advertising by the food and restaurant industries is again in the numbers. In most cases, carbohydrates are being replaced by fat. (Remember seeing the Atkins friendly signs at a host of eateries?) Remember, a gram of fat is worth nearly twice the amount of calories as a gram of carbohydrate. To make matters worse, all fats ARE NOT REALLY created equal. If the substitution for carbs is olive oil or omega-3 fats (fish), the exchange can be beneficial. Unfortunately, often the reality is hydrogenated or trans fats find their way into the foods (see the nutrition section for additional information).

Doctor—Patient Partnerships

- The current "Doctor—Patient Relationship" does not encourage adequate patient input.
- Developing a "Doctor—Patient Partnership" encourages the patient to actively participate in the healing process. This requires the medical provider to "hear" and communicate with you. It requires you to be accountable for your health-related actions and activities.
- Partnership type communication will sustain one through the trying times of healing.

Due to changes that have taken place over the last 10 to 15 years within managed healthcare, patients have become aware of a decrease in quantity face-to-face time with their doctor. Unfortunately, this is perceived as a decrease in quality of medical service. It is important to understand how the "business" of healthcare has changed. As an example, when I started in practice in 1980, physicians were paid "fee for service." The physician provided a service and was compensated for the time it took to deal with the patient's problem. Each procedure completed is coded so that there is a continuity of understanding between the physician's office and the party responsible for reimbursement. Office visits range from brief to complex depending on a number of variable factors, including time. Prior to changes of the last decade, physicians billed depending upon the level of service provided. If a procedure was brief the office visit was billed at the lowest reimbursement. On the other hand, if the patient had complex issues in which the physician had to order tests, review records, consult, examine, and develop a treatment plan, this qualified at one of the higher levels of service. Under managed healthcare, an office visit is just that, an office visit. It doesn't make any difference whether the amount of time spent with a patient is 2 minutes or 20 minutes; the reimbursement, in dollars, from the insurance carrier is the same.

A true story of one of my patients reflects this problem. She came in frustrated, saying that she had the same primary care physician for 15 years but wanted the name of a new doctor. When I inquired why, she stated that when she called to set up an appointment she told the receptionist that she had a number of issues to discuss with the doctor. She was informed that she could be seen for only one condition and would have to make additional appointments if she needed to address the others. Unfortunately, I am sure many of you have had a similar experience. In many cases, today's doctor has lost the ability to meet a patient's total needs. Physicians have to focus on the most pressing need. As patients are aware, this has led to the use ancillary personnel, nurse practitioners and physician assistants, to deal with all but the most pressing or complex issues. This example is given to illustrate the need for doctor/patient partnerships. In a partnership it is essential that both individuals bring something to the table. The patient, when possible, needs to research their condition. Understanding that medicine is complex, there are many good resources available, including utilizing the Internet and library. A basic understanding allows you to control the conversation by bringing the doctor back to your main concern.

A patient goes to the doctor seeking to know four things: what is their problem; can the doctor fix it; how long is it going to take; and what is it going to cost. When the patient has familiarized themselves with their problem, the explanation of the condition and treatment options will make more sense. This assumes that you have an idea of what your condition is. If you do not have a name for your condition or a general idea how to research it, you may have to wait until after the initial visit with the doctor to delve deeper. At the least, go to the doctor knowing that you need to address the four areas of concern. Often, patients will leave the doctor's office without a clear idea of what the problem is, what needs to be done with regard to the treatment program, or without an understanding of what to expect in the following days or weeks. Physicians need to be held accountable. Adequately fulfilling the patients' expectations makes them a better physician. A patient, who can help control the conversation, will make sure the doctor addresses their concerns. Patients, in healthcare today, are too passive. They have a right and an obligation to expect a working doctor/patient partnership.

When you are with the doctor, let them know by your attitude and attention that you are interested in regaining health. Often, you may not remember the things you wished to discuss with him/her. Write a list and prioritize it. Pick 2 or 3 things that are important. Take notes so that once you have talked to the doctor, you remember what was said. If problems arise after a visit, ask for a copy of your records. The new HIPPA regulations allow you to have a copy of your chart. (If you want a copy of your entire chart, be prepared to pay a reasonable copying fee.) Once you have an idea of what the problem is, do research before the next doctor's visit. By following these recommendations, you will have demonstrated interest in being compliant and to do your part in getting well. This will assist in fulfilling your part of the doctor-patient partnership.

The ABCs

ABC stands for ABOUT BEING COMPLETE. ABOUT is the recognition that individual healthcare is about you. While that may sound obvious, the fact is that women by nature are nurturers, and in their nurturing they tend to overlook their personal healthcare needs. The idea that it is about you has a certain selfish ring to it. Understand that taking care of oneself is not a selfish act, but actually leads to an improved ability to nurture. When you are healthy, the ability to nurture comes from the overflow of wellness. Think of the body as a goblet. When filled with nourishment it will overflow to others. If the goblet is nearly empty, there is little to pour into the lives of others.

The B in ABC is for BEING. It is the ability to live in today. Of all things, I find this the most difficult to explain, and the most difficult to live out. BEING acknowledges the ability to eliminate fear if the future and/or the burden of guilt and pain of the past. This is an important part of mental wellness and, in my opinion, rests on a spiritual foundation. Encompassed in the idea of BEING is the reality that you are not responsible for other people's actions. You are responsible for your reactions to the various situations in life. I like to say that life is what happens while you're planning something else. How you react to those something else's in life is a good indicator of your ability to live in the present. At a deeper level, it reveals the degree of satisfaction and peace within your life. There was once a philosopher that put the following on his answering machine—"Who are you, and what do you want?" If you think these questions to be superficial; most people go through life without asking!

The final part of ABC is C. C stands for COMPLETE. Total healthcare is not just a physical reality but dependent upon the mind, the body, and the spirit. Think of it as a 3-legged stool. Each leg is dependent on and to the other legs. Excellent research over the last decade has shown that every cell of our body is capable of feeling and therefore intimately related to non-conscious activity of the brain. Our perceptions, expectations, and spiritual awareness all affect and are effected by total body cellular activity. A deficit in 1 of the 3 areas will ultimately have a detrimental affect on the other two. Unfortunately, we are not aware of the destructive processes going on inside our bodies, as they may not immediately result in symptoms. Remember the previously stated goal—to regain health and wellness, not remove symptoms. A step in that direction requires that you embrace the ABCs.

You Are Not a Captive of Your Genes

The Role of Integrative/Functional Medicine

Integrative/functional medicine is the based on the awareness of the interrelatedness of bodily systems. It includes nutrition tailored to the individual, the substantial distinction between genetic disposition (suggesting a fatalism) and genetic expression (modifiable). It is the clinical discipline designed to promote health, anticipate and prevent disease, and correct existing disease and dysfunction. This is accomplished by improving physiological function. The primary focus is on the functional integrity of the body's metabolic systems. There are two types of aging: metabolic and genetic. Lifestyle changes can prevent accelerated metabolic aging. The same lifestyle changes may slow or eliminate the expression of genetic aging. Your genetics may "load the gun," but it is lifestyle that "pulls the trigger."

The chart below represents the impact of lifestyle choices coupled with genetic predisposition. The worst-case scenario combines "bad" genes contributed by both parents and "bad" lifestyle choices. As expected, the individuals risk factors, *i.e.* depreciating health, are high. Because lifestyle represents the modifiable part of this equation, the risk can be elevated to a medium level with the application of positive change.

Genes	Genes	Lifestyle	Risk
Mom	Dad	Good Bad	Low Med High
Good	Good	Good	Low
Good	Good	Bad	Med to High
Good	Bad	Good	Med
Good	Bad	Bad	High
Bad	Good	Good	Med
Bad	Good	Bad	High
Bad	Bad	Good	Med
Bad	Bad	Bad	High

How does this apply to you? Consider the blood work done at your annual physical. The clinical lab values of these tests are ranges considered compatible with life and are generally rather wide. They do not necessarily reflect desired values consistent with optimal health. In reality, the number of tests included in your annual evaluation has progressively decreased over the last decade. Insurance reimbursement generally dictates the number of tests allowed and does not equate with the ability to effectively monitor metabolic function. Functional laboratory testing includes a larger number of tested items and presents with a narrower range of acceptable values (see below examples). These test values allow your physician to design a program tailored to your specific metabolic needs. Look for a partnership with a physician who understands the value of functional testing. For more information on the practical application of a functional/integrative approach to your healthcare see "Food As Medicine" and "Part 6 - How This Applies to You."

Example of Clinical vs. Functional Lab Value

LAB TEST	CLINICAL VALUE	FUNCTIONAL VALUE
GLUCOSE	65 – 100	75 - 93
CALCIUM	8.5 – 10.6	9.4 – 9.8
PROTEIN, TOTAL	6 –8.5	7 – 7.2
SODIUM	135 - 148	140 - 142

Step by Step

Learn—Commit—Apply—Improve

In order to be successful in your quest for health and wellness, you must have a realistic, workable plan. There are two parts to this plan. The first is to "plan your work"; the second is to "work your plan." Please note the specific order to this. It is about having a fail-proof system. I would encourage you to read Dr. Phil McGraw's recent book, *The Ultimate Weight Solution*, to understand the seven steps he recommends for building this system. For now, do your research, "your homework." Before the actual application, make a "conscious" commitment to the goal. Once you have finished the CD and/or text, you will make a "written" commitment. Each section has practical applications, and I want you to write down 1 or 2 from each area (this is the beginning of Progressive Practical Application). Find yourself an accountability partner—someone who understands your goals and will encourage you during frustrating times. Again, this is the reason for having a physician who is in partnership with you. Application includes the new things you will do and the old things you will not do. To aid in your success, I would encourage you to "clean up" your personal environment. Remove or discontinue the things that are a hindrance to you. This may include foods, cosmetics, social activities, and in some cases, acquaintances. The end result of your learning, commitment, and effective application will be improved health and wellness.

A Paradigm Shift

Babbling Brook to Rushing River

The healthcare system is complex; and, for the most part, modern healthcare has failed the patient, especially women. A better term for the healthcare system we have today is a *rescue system*. Little emphasis is placed on prevention while significant amounts of money and research have gone to "rescue and repair."

The "babbling brook to rushing river" analogy will emphasize to you the importance of: 1) prioritizing healthcare decisions and maximizing choices (picking the area for initial change that will have the greatest impact on overall healthcare), and 2) the nature of preventative care. This is especially true for parents in developing positive health habits and lifestyle choices for their children.

In a visual picture, see a group of rocks from which water is flowing. As it starts down the mountain, see the beginning a babbling brook of pure, clear water. As the brook travels farther down the mountain it begins to pick up speed and grow in size. When the stream gets to the bottom of the mountain, it has now become deeper and wider, and the water is flowing swiftly. Here is the second half of our picture. Now we have a rushing river.

Picture the small brook traveling down the mountainside, ever increasing in size, speed, and volume. In a healthcare context, equate evaluating your health status to checking water quality of the stream. The closer to the source, the easier it is to check: the farther downstream the more difficult. The nearer to the source, the less likely the stream is to be polluted and if needed the easier to clean up. As you travel downstream, there are more opportunities to contaminate the waters. Because the river is now wider and deeper, the more difficult it will be to evaluate and clean.

There are two applications of this analogy. The earlier (nearer the source of the stream) you understand the importance of your health related decisions, the easier to have positive effects on the remainder of your life. This is especially true concerning the decisions made for your children, and the mentoring effects of personal choices. The war on cancer is a perfect example of this concept in action. Since the National Cancer Act was enacted in 1971, the annual death rate has increased by 73%—over one and a half times as fast as the population growth (the death rate over a 14-month period in 2004-2005 is estimated at 563,700—more than the combined war deaths of all of America's wars!) Most advances, with regard to actual treatment (drugs and surgery), are associated with a handful of less common malignancies: Hodgkin's disease, leukemia, childhood cancers, and cancer of the testes and thyroid. Thirty-three years ago, the 5-year survival rate was just over 50%; today it is estimated at 63%. Concern exists that these modest gains are not from ongoing research (and the major funding to the National Cancer Institute and other research centers), but primarily from lifestyle factors. These behavioral changes include: quitting smoking, earlier detection of breast cancer resulting from mammography and breast self-exam, and current screening methods for prostate and colon cancer. Ruth Etzioni, at Seattle's Fred Hutchinson Cancer Research Center, notes that the long-term (5-year) survival rate for breast, colon, and lung cancer, once it has metastasized, has not significantly improved over the last 33 years.

For many years, the focus of medical care for the major diseases has been directed to conquering the disease in its late stages (rescue medicine). A mindset change with regard to some cancers and heart disease has resulted in earlier detection and treatment, but the greater majority of money and research remains directed to the former (generally unsuccessful) paradigm. An example of a positive change in the research process is current research into the relationship of cancer growth and angiogenesis (the development of new blood vessels needed to feed the growth of a cancer). There are currently over 40 drugs in clinical trials associated with retarding or eliminating the blood supply to cancerous growths. The sad side to this "recent" development is that Judah Folkman, M.D., first pioneered it over 43 years ago. The major institutes and research facilities rejected this direction of treatment and continued to attack cancer in the latter stages. The mindset was, cure cancer once diagnosed, not prevent it from developing in the first place. Even today, the application of this treatment protocol is not being effectively utilized. In keeping with the old mindset of "cure," it is being tested on patients with advanced staged cancer, not at the first appearance of cancer markers. The greatest success will come when the medical community accepts the challenge to treat at the "babbling brook" end of the process. When science develops reliable early indicators (protein markers), coupled with lifestyle changes, and drugs (when needed), we will finally be able to say we are gaining in our quest to "win the war" against cancer and other debilitating diseases.

The second application: discovering (learn and commit) and applying those health related habits that will have the greatest affect. Stopping eating "super-sized" portions is an excellent improvement, but stopping smoking is even better. When you start on the road to health choose those areas that will give you the greatest return for your investment of time, money, effort, etc. One change upstream will have a greater effect on the water (your health) downstream than a number of changes at the mid-point or beyond.

These two applications are particularly relevant to understanding the devastating effect stress has on the body. The goal is to have you implement at least one change in each of the four focus areas: 1) stress reduction; 2) exposure to environmental estrogens and toxins; 3) exposure to prescription estrogens; and 4) proper nourishment and nutrition. If you can make just one change initially, reduce stress!

Part Three

Stress Reduction

The symptoms and the illness are not the same thing. The illness exists long before the symptoms. Rather than being the illness, the symptoms are the beginning of its cures. The fact that they are unwanted makes them all the more a phenomenon of grace—a gift of God, a message from the unconscious, if you will, to invite self-examination and repair.
—M. Scott Peck, *The Road Less Traveled*

An Overview

Stress is a reality of life. Our goal is not to eliminate stress, but to balance it. There are 2 types of stress: 1) acute, life threatening and 2) chronic, non-life threatening. Chronic stress can be either from too much of a pleasurable activity or from day-after-day exposure to noxious activities, chemicals, or lifestyle. From a physiological standpoint, the body cannot tell the difference. Chronic stress results in an abnormal production of the stress hormones, adrenaline and cortisol (produced in the adrenal glands). It affects the production of insulin (produced in the pancreas) and the body's response to carbohydrates (sugar). All three of these hormones affect the balance or activity of thyroid hormone, estrogen, progesterone, and testosterone. Symptoms related to chronic stress include adrenal exhaustion (you get extremely tired/fatigued in the p.m.), fibromyalgia, depression, increased degenerative diseases/arthritis, suppressed immune system, and irritable bowel syndrome. Symptoms related to chronic insulin production include hypoglycemia, Syndrome X/insulin resistance syndrome, elevated cholesterol and triglycerides, increased abdominal fat storage, fatigue, insomnia, fuzzy thinking, and irregular menstrual cycles. Two end result conditions related to altered insulin production are "Adult Onset Diabetes—Type II" and increased cardiovascular disease. The last is termed "ischemic heart disease" in females and is a leading cause of death in women over the age of 60.

The Details

Adrenalin and Cortisol

An overview of the function of these hormones is in order. Adrenalin, or epinephrine and cortisol are both hormones produced in your adrenal glands. Adrenalin is the fight-or-flight hormone. When you are scared your heart pounds, blood will rush to your brain, and the larger muscles in your arms and legs help you move. Your pupils dilate. Under the right circumstances, this is the hormone that can save your life. The problem is the body does not know the difference between perceived danger and real danger. It cannot differentiate between circumstances that are life threatening versus ones that are chronic and non-life threatening. Recurrent stressful daily activities begin to cause a phenomenon entitled "entraining." The subconscious becomes used to the stimuli and automatically responds even with a minor perceived stress.

Cortisol has a major effect on cellular metabolism, muscle tissue maintenance, suppression of inflammation, as well as maintaining sugar levels in the brain. The latter is accomplished by affecting liver function in the conversion of sugar and the production of cholesterol.

Two areas in the brain control the majority of hormonal activity: (1) the hypothalamus, which communicates with (2) the pituitary gland, that, in turn directs hormonal production. There is a "negative feedback loop" that allows the body to monitor how much of a hormone is being produced; and when the level goes up, it tells the pituitary gland to turn the production down, and visa versa.

Remember, none of the hormones operate independently and each one has an intimate affect on the balance of the other hormones. A prime example of this is understanding that your cortisol production is at its highest in the morning and tapers off towards midnight. As long as the levels and the timing are maintained correctly, the other hormones have an opportunity to remain in balance. With chronic production of cortisol, especially when you have levels that are lower in the morning and build towards the afternoon, the pancreas secretes increased levels of insulin. This may ultimately progress to insulin resistance—"Syndrome X"/"metabolic syndrome." The body perceives this behavior as a situation where food may be in short supply.

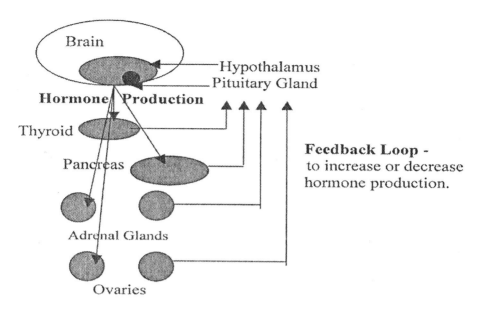

The end result is storage of fat in the abdomen. A final consequence of these physiological actions may be adult onset diabetes (Type II). Cortisol will also decrease thyroid sensitivity. The individual who has symptoms suggestive of low thyroid production may evidence this.

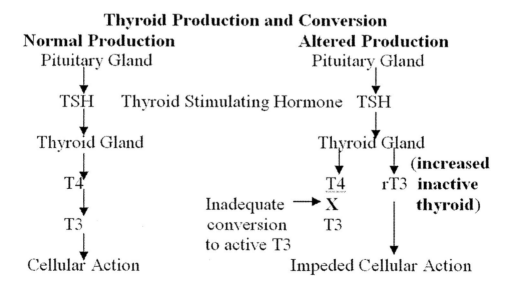

The standard lab test for thyroid function is called TSH (thyroid stimulating hormone). The test results may appear normal but you continue to experience symptoms. This is because the body is producing a normal amount of thyroid (inactive T4), that it is not effectively being converted to the active form (T3). (See above figure). Supplementation with Synthroid without correcting a cortisol deficiency will not result in improved function or energy levels. Additional tests, including reverse T3 (rT3—an inactive form as a result of inadequate conversion of T4 to T3) and a.m. and p.m. cortisol levels, will help to clarify this problem. Adrenal exhaustion, the end result of chronic stress and cortisol production, may warrant short-term supplementation with hydrocortisone. Again, it must be emphasized that the goal is to simulate the body's normal physiological level of cortisol (as with every other hormone where supplementation is recommended). Cortisol supplementation should be monitored with 24-hour urine levels of hydrocortisone output.

24-Hour Cortisol Production

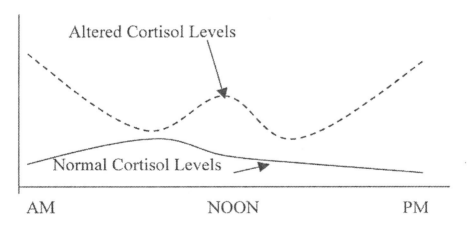

I have noted that cortisol is important in maintaining brain function through the regulation of blood sugar in the form of glucose. Chronic exposure to cortisol kills brain cells, especially in the areas associated with memory. I believe that excess levels of cortisol are responsible for what fibromyalgia patients refer to as "fibro fog," a dullness of brain function. There is a relationship between appropriate cortisol levels and bone production. When bone is exposed to chronic levels of cortisol, there is altered bone metabolism (bone build-up versus bone break-down). Excess cortisol results in increased deposition of abdominal fat and poor fat metabolism as a result of altered thyroid function and conversion. Cellular receptor sites may be up-regulated (increased sensitivity) or down-regulated (decreased sensitivity) in the presence of cortisol. An increase of estrogen sensitivity may be accompanied by an increase of conversion of progesterone to estrogen. Progesterone is a precursor to the other sex hormones, and this conversion results in an imbalance and increased estrogen dominance.

Chronic Exposure to Cortisol

- Kills brain cells
- Dulls brain function—"fibro-fog"
- Decreases bone density
- Increases abdominal fat
- Increases estrogen receptor cell sensitivity
- Increases estrogen dominance
- Decreases immune response

Finally, there is a decrease in immune response. We are all probably aware of and have experienced this. When under a stressful situation, about the time the stress eases up, the next thing that happens is you get a viral infection—a cold. Current scientific research notes that, not just situations we perceive as stressful, but every thought produces neurologic and immunologic responses.

Bruce McEwen, author of *The End of Stress As We Know It* and head of the neuroendocrinology lab at Rockefeller University of New York, highlighted the end result of chronic stress. He confirmed that the body could not tell the difference between real or perceived stress. No matter the cause, the physiological responses were the same. After an initial surge of cortisol, the body went through the process of calming down. Repeated daily trips, up-and-down "this mountain," resulted in the above noted destructive actions.

Adrenalin and cortisol are produced in different areas of the adrenal glands. The end result of chronically elevated levels of these may lead to adrenal exhaustion. There are pathological reasons for increased or decreased levels of both these hormones, but they are relatively rare. The typical cause for altered adrenal function is related to lifestyle choices.

The role of insulin and the associated concerns related to excess production will be discussed under the nutrition section.

Practical Stress Reduction

Lifestyle changes that will balance stress and therefore your hormones include:

· Understanding that "unproductive time" is not wasted time.
· Downtime is necessary for the body to heal –schedule daily "downtime."
· Make a "what irritates me" list and explore alternate ways to react to them.
· Take a "news holiday"—start by turning off the television and/or do not read a newspaper for 1 day per week.
· Prioritize your activities—make a "to do list" and set realistic goals.
· Organize your personal work environment at home and at the office.
· Pick your battles carefully (especially with your kids)—remember the goal is to win the war and not every battle.
· If you feel totally overwhelmed, ask for help, including professional counseling.

Relaxation Exercise: Lie on your back with a pillow under your knees to relax the lower back. Breathe "in" and at the same time push your stomach out (this pulls your diaphragm down drawing air into your lungs). Breathe "in" to the count of 1-2. Breathe "out" as your stomach is pulled in (flattened). Count 1-2-3-4 as you breathe "out." Repeat this exercise daily for 5-15 minutes (as time allows). After a while, you will not have to count to maintain the rhythm. Start to "listen" to your breath as it goes in and out. You are beginning to train your body to RELAX, and it will soon associate the sound of your breath with a new pattern of relaxation.

Exercise—An Overview

Cardiovascular: The goal is to get your heart rate up into what is referred to as the "training zone." The target range or "training zone" is determined by taking 220, subtracting your age, and for women, multiplying it by 0.7 and men 0.8. (This will vary by the text that you read, but generally this is a conservative training zone.) Your goal is to get to that rate and maintain it for a 20 to 30 minute period, followed by a 5 minute cool down. Try doing this 2 to 3 days a week. Combine this with 1 or 2 days of light comfortable walking for 30 to 45 minutes. To facilitate weight loss, the National Heart, Lung, and Blood Institute recommends at least 30 minutes of moderate exercise 5 days per week. (In a recent abstract that sited the "1998 National Health Interview Survey," only 54% of women using exercise as part of a weight-loss strategy met the minimum recommendation.) When walking at a comfortable pace, let your arms swing freely by your sides. Bending the elbows and pumping will tighten and stress the shoulder and neck muscles. For individuals with low back problems, I recommend that you complete your walks on relatively flat surfaces. Walking in your neighborhood may be too hilly. If it is, try going to one of the schools with a track or use the mall before opening hours. Many of the malls have designated measured walking areas. If you have ankle, knee, or sacral problems, do not walk or run on the pavement at the side of the road. Most roads have a crown (they are higher at the middle and lower at the sides), which causes a postural imbalance when walking on the sides. In effect, you are walking with one leg higher than the other. While doing this occasionally is not generally dangerous, it is the repetition that leads to problems. This is a good time to mention the importance of varying your workouts. In addition to avoiding boredom, it helps exercise different muscle groups. If you exercise at the gym, utilize different pieces of cardiovascular equipment on different days. If you walk outside, one-day walk in one direction in your neighborhood, then change your route. Try the track or the mall on a third day, and then start the cycle over.

Posture: Ideal posture would be picturing a plumb-line that passes through the middle of the ear, the middle of the shoulder and hip bone, just behind the knee and though the middle of the ankle bone. Most individuals, especially women, have poor upper body posture. The condition is associated with a head forward position (especially when seated), slumped/rounded shoulders, and a flattening or caving in of the chest. This posture is made worse by extended periods of computer data entry (and other jobs that require you to sit and look down for long periods), tall thin women, and women with large breasts. I jokingly tell my female patients that the worst job, from a postural standpoint, is a 6-foot woman, with large breasts, who teaches computer to first graders. Other concerns that tend to contribute to poor posture are nursing mothers and mothers of preschoolers. Both of these activities require long periods of time bending forward and looking down, thus rounding the shoulders. Symptoms, related to poor upper body posture, include tingling in the hands and fingers. This particular posture may lead to a condition called functional thoracic outlet syndrome (TOS). Individuals with TOS tend to have a greater incidence of carpal tunnel syndrome. Surgical release of carpal tunnel syndrome, without properly addressing the presence of TOS, will result in a poor outcome. If you are awakening with your hands asleep (tingling) and/or your hands tingle when they are on the steering wheel or above your head, you need to be evaluated for TOS. Strictly adhering to the noted postural correction exercises below will eliminate or reduce the symptoms. Once you have worked to improve your posture, maintaining it becomes a lifetime commitment. I would like to see the following exercises attached to every bra sold. Developing females (adolescent) need to be convinced of the importance of upper body posture. This is one of those measures where an ounce of prevention is worth a pound of cure.

I recommend two exercises to help postural alignment:

1. "Shoulder Rolls": Start by sitting erect and bringing the shoulders up toward the ears. At the top of the motion start to roll the shoulders backward and at the same time press the chest forward. Continue to bring the shoulders down and back to the starting position. Do 10 repetitions each to a count of 1-2-3-4. Up-1, back-2, down-3, and return to the start position-4. This exercise should be done 5 times per day: first time you are in the bathroom to shower or put on make-up, mid-morning, lunch, mid-afternoon, and the last time in the bathroom to shower or take off make-up. For individuals who have difficulty or discomfort with shoulder rolls, the same benefit can be achieved by doing corner stretches.

"Corner stretches": I call this exercise "timeout for adults." Start by standing 1 arm's length from a corner of a room. Place each hand, about shoulder height, about 18 inches from the corner—you will have one hand on each side of the wall coming out of the corner. Lean forward like you are trying to touch your nose in the corner. Go as far as you are comfortable—you should feel a stretch in the front of your shoulders and chest. Once you have gone as far as you can, look up toward the ceiling—this increases the stretch in the upper chest. Hold the position for 15 to 30 seconds and return to the starting position. Relax and then repeat the exercise 3 to 5 times. Try doing this 3 times per day—morning, noon, and night.

2. The second exercise is completed while taking those recommended walks. During the walk, concentrate on tightening the abdominal muscles—pull your bellybutton back toward your spine. This will cause the oblique abdominal muscles to tighten, flattening the lower tummy and strengthening the low back. I find this exercise helpful for most individuals for a number of reasons: 1) the oblique abdominals are major contributors to low back stability, and most individuals will not or cannot complete enough oblique crunches to properly strengthen them; 2) because it is done in association with walking, there is a greater chance for compliance. Crunches too often exacerbate low back and neck problems that lead to inconsistent follow through. While you may not develop a "six-pack" (marked definition of the abdominal muscles), you will improve total body posture as well as help strengthen the back.

These two exercises, together, will make a dramatic improvement in posture and will have a positive affect on low back and neck problems.

Bra selection: An aspect related to exercise is protecting your body from injury secondary to repetitive motion. The selection of the proper type and fit of bra is an extremely important issue associated with repetitive stress. The first area to address is the type of bra: either compression or encapsulation. The best way to describe a compression bra is to think pancakes. The bra compresses the breast tissue against the chest and ribcage, thus minimizing movement. The downside is primarily aesthetic, the "uni-breast" look. The encapsulation type bra is one that supports each breast separately. This can be a better choice for women with breast sizes DD or above. There are bras that provide aspects of each. The type of activity that a woman engages in will assist in determining the amount of support necessary. A sports bra that provides twice the support of a regular bra may be adequate for weight workouts. More support is needed when cardiovascular activities are added that result in bouncing of the breast. There are various materials of bra construction, cotton, Lycra/Spandex, nylon microfiber, including those for wicking sweat (moisture management - Coolmax). Once you have determined a type, the most important aspect is the fit. The material of the bra should lie smoothly, the chest band snug but not too tight, and the shoulder straps should not pull or bind. I recommend that at some time a woman have a professional fit her "everyday" bras. With regard to sports bras, try those with as wide of straps and chest band as reasonably comfortable. The compression of the breast tissue across the chest, in association with wider shoulder straps, will decrease the pressure on the upper trapezius/shoulder-to-neck muscles. When there is less weight "pulling down" on the front of the chest, there will be less strain on the neck and mid to upper back muscles. A properly fitting bra, both regular and sports, is an important part of achieving and maintaining improved posture.

Stretching: Before any exercise, it is important to warm up and make stretching a part of the routine. It needs to be done in that order. It is much easier to stretch a muscle, which has been warmed up, so I highly encourage each person to walk for about 5 minutes at a leisurely pace and then do stretching.

If you are at home or in the gym doing exercise, complete about 5 minutes on a treadmill or one of the other types of aerobic equipment. Get off, stretch the low back, the front and back of the legs, the front and back of the arms and shoulders, and the neck. Return to your exercise, whether it is continuing the cardiovascular, an aerobic exercise, or starting weight training. As mentioned earlier, some form of weight training is important for all women because of the osteoporosis aspect. Recent research has also related consistent exercise with improved cognitive function in postmenopausal women. What was interesting was the fact that the benefits did not differ whether the exercise was moderate or vigorous. Therefore, this can be accomplished using light hand weights (3 and 5 pound). These can be purchased at super stores or specialty sports shops. If you are working out at the gym, I encourage you to work with a trainer, at least for the first few weeks, so that you understand the importance of body mechanics. Learn the correct positions for utilizing the free weights and exercise machines. Nothing will stop continuing your exercise faster than injury. A good rule associated with weight lifting is to keep your head up, in a "neutral posture." During any exercise in which you see yourself, eyeball-to-eyeball, in a mirror, maintain the visual contact throughout the exercise. If you are not in a room with a mirror, pick a spot on the wall, eye height from the floor, and stare at it while exercising. This will reduce injuries to the neck and upper back regions.

A Home Exercise Program

A basic understanding of a few exercise terms will help you get started. Muscles move all of our body parts from small (fingers and toes) to large (arms, legs, and torso). Generally, muscles are balanced, a set on one side and a set on the other side of a joint. These move the structures back and forth. The goal of a well-designed program is to balance the workout to include the muscles of upper body (back, chest, arms, and shoulders) and lower body (legs, thighs, hips, and buttocks) and those on the front and backside of the body. Exercises are grouped into "reps" (repetitions—the number of times you complete a particular exercise) and "sets (the number of times that you do the repetitions). Example: 8 reps for 3 sets—you will do the exercise 8 times (you have completed 1 set), rest for a minute or two and then do 8 more repetitions (completion of the 2nd set). After another short rest, the final set will be completed. It is now time to start another exercise. Try to work the muscles on opposite sides of a joint—example: biceps (the muscles on the front of the arm that bend the forearm at the elbow) and triceps (the muscles on the back of the arm that straighten the forearm at the elbow).

A balanced program can be complete with a set of light hand weights and rubber/elastic tubing (Therabands).

Upper Body:

- Biceps: Either standing or seated, start with the weights in your hands down at your sides. Slowly bend your arm at the elbow and lower it back down to the starting position. Repeat with the other arm. Follow the above-recommended repetitions (8) for either 2 or 3 sets. Start with the lightest weight that you feel comfortable with and gradually increase. You will know it is OK to increase the weight when you can complete all 3 sets with out difficulty. *Remember to keep the head up; do not look down at your hands while exercising!*
- Triceps: Sitting in a chair raise one arm straight above the head with your palms facing inward. Lower the weight behind your head and then straighten it back out. Do not completely straighten the arm each time as this may irritate the elbow region.

- Shoulders: Starting with a light weight in each hand. Stand with the palms facing backward. Raise each arm (straight) one at a time from the side, straight ahead until it is shoulder height. Lower it to the side and repeat with the other arm. The outer sides of the shoulders can be exercised by starting with the palms facing the body and raising both arms together away from the body to just below shoulder level (think of making a snow angel).
- Chest: Bench presses can be completed lying on your back on a short bench or ottoman. Start with the weights in your hands, palms facing toward your feet, resting next to your chest. This exercise can also be completed with the palms facing inward. Raise both arms straight above your body, and then return them down next to the chest.

Lower Body:

- Buttocks and thighs: Lunges should initially be done without weights. Once you feel comfortable and balanced slowly add weight. From a standing position step forward with the right foot about 18 inches. Bend the knees until the left knee nearly touches the floor then straighten up and bring the right foot back next to the left. Repeat stepping forward with the left foot and bringing the right knee near the floor. This is one repetition for each leg.
- Calves: Calf raises can be completed either on the flat floor or for more difficulty on the edge of a step or flat board. Starting with the feet flat on the floor raise up on your toes, hold for a count of 2 or 3 and lower back down. Doing this exercise on a step or board will help to stretch the Achilles tendon, which tends to become short and tight from a woman's higher heeled shoes.

This basic workout should take about 30 minutes to complete. Warm up for 5 minutes prior to starting by walking inside or outside. Complete the weight workout 2 days per week. Engage in a 30-minute cardiovascular exercise (walking, jogging, bike, or elliptical trainer) on 3 other days of the week. All of these are "weight bearing exercise" and are an important component for strengthening the bones of the hips and spine.

In our busy work-a-day world, you may feel like you do not have 30 minutes, 5 times a week, to dedicate to exercise. A little creative time management will allow you to gain most of the benefits by completing the exercises in segments or intervals. If you only have 10 or 15 minutes each morning or evening, do either upper or lower body weight work—not both. Try the upper body on Monday and Thursday and the lower body on Tuesday and Friday. Try walking for 15 minutes at lunch and park farther from your office. Remember our goal is health as a result of lifestyle changes; take the stairs not the elevator or escalator; park at the one end of the mall and walk briskly to the other.

Chiropractic

Chiropractic is the fastest growing of the complementary medical disciplines. It is based on the philosophy that an intact nervous system, free from interference by structural misalignment, will increase the body's capacity to function efficiently. It is common that people associate chiropractors with neck and back pain. While this is generally the majority of what the average chiropractor sees during a workday, it is far from the real scope that chiropractic can affect. When the body is structurally aligned, there is a reduction in mechanical stress to the joints, muscles, tendons, and ligaments. Increased stress in these areas generally leads to tissue destruction and associated inflammation. Once this process has begun, the body must respond by activating the proper hormones to deal with the injury. While not detrimental to the body when this happens on an occasional basis, it is the chronic presence of tissue destruction that results in hormonal imbalance. On a cellular basis, it is important that each cell receive clear nerve innervation to function and replicate as designed. Chiropractic is effective as a preventative measure when initiated in childhood and adolescence. Recent studies have validated the effectiveness of chiropractic in dealing with recurrent ear infections and colic in children. Returning to the stream analogy, this represents *cleaning up the stream* near its origin where a small change may have greater affect.

Practical Application

- Practice a form of "stress reduction" on a daily basis—see "Practical Stress Reduction."
- Stretch daily—there are a number of good VHS tapes available with instruction. I particularly like using an exercise ball for stretching.
- Walk 3-4 days per week for 15 to 45 minutes. Try to reach your training zone at least 2 days per week.
- Lift weights 2 days per week—see "A Home Exercise Program."
- Receive regular chiropractic care.

Part Four

Environmental Estrogens

Someday they will make one tombstone for housewives everywhere with a standard inscription. It will read, "I told you I was sick."
—Erma Bombeckm, *At Wits End*

An Overview

"Better Living Through Chemistry" was a popular slogan a few decades ago. Unfortunately, this chemistry brings you in constant contact with potentially dangerous chemicals found in cleaning products, plastics, soaps, pesticides, paint, carpet, cosmetics, and foodstuffs. You need to become aware of what you put "on and in" your bodies. The end result of chronic exposure to these products is a condition termed "estrogen dominance" and "endocrine disruption." Estrogen dominance is a relative increase of estrogen and estrogen-like metabolic activity to the amount of progesterone activity in the body (see Part 5—How This Applies to You). Chemicals that cause abnormal endocrine/hormonal activity (not just estrogen) are termed endocrine disruptors (ED).

The focus of this section is on the effects of environmental estrogens, estrogen-like substances, and endocrine disruptors. The contents cover material that is not universally agreed upon in the scientific community. There are contradictory opinions regarding the long-term effects of both environmental estrogen (and estrogen-like products) and prescription estrogen hormone replacement on the human body. While there is strong evidence supporting abnormal growth and genetic change among exposed animals, scientists have not been quick to equate similar exposures as a risk for people. Because of the potential for genetic damage that may be passed to subsequent generations, I believe that it wise to err on the side of concern and protection.

Protecting oneself starts with learning to be a label reader. That said, it is nearly impossible to understand what you find listed on the products you purchase. Later in this section, I am going to give a list of the common chemicals found in food and cosmetics. You need to know about these because, in some cases, exposure to individual chemicals may be detrimental; in others, the cumulative affect of multiple chemicals or repeated exposure may result is serious cellular damage and health consequences.

Xenoestrogens and Cellular Function

Every man, woman, and child living in an industrialized country is virtually swimming in a sea of environmental chemical waste. A great deal of this is the result of petrochemicals (the refinement of crude oil), the use of pesticides, and chemical treatment of our foods. This includes estrogen given to livestock and chickens to add weight and antibiotics to fend off disease in the close quarters of animals raised for food. Collectively, these chemicals are called xenoestrogens or xenobiotics. If you find these terms unfamiliar and strange, it is because that is exactly what they are. The prefix "xeno" is Greek for foreign or strange. Xenoestrogens and xenobiotics are by-products of industrial and chemical processing. One of their dangers lies in their ability to mimic the activity and affects of natural estrogen. Additionally, they can affect a cell's ability to reproduce itself, damage DNA, and/or up-regulate (increase) or down-regulate (decrease) hormonal function.

A basic understanding of how this happens is in order. While many of these foreign chemicals are not actually estrogen, they tend to bind to cells preferentially (for an unknown reason the foreign chemical will fill the receptor site first). It was once believed that cellular activity was triggered when cellular receptor sites (picture them as a lock) were stimulated by an exact hormone or chemical (pictured as keys). In reality, the cellular receptors are not as particular as previously thought, and various similar substances may bind to the receptors. Once the fraudulent "key" binds to a cellular "lock" (we are going to use estrogen receptors as our example), a number of possible effects result. In the above figure the estrogen and xenoestrogen molecules have similarly sized binding properties, where

Circulating estrogen molecules

Binding site for estrogen

Cellular receptor site

Xenoestrogen may bind preferentially

Cellular Actions

either will fit into the cell's receptor site. Note that the xenoestrogen has an additional property attached that will result in altered cellular actions. By filling the receptor site (the lock is full), it prevents the body's natural circulating estrogen from binding. This may in turn result in the body decreasing its production of natural estrogen. Finally, this preferential binding may cause cellular actions (turning on or off biochemical pathways) that are not the same as those resulting from binding with natural estrogen. These abnormal cellular activities, ultimately, are passed on to the next generation of cells when the abnormal cells divide.

All of the sex hormones (steroid hormones) are derived from cholesterol. Estrogen has a distinct structure from the other steroid hormones called a phenolated A-ring (a part of the cholesterol framework). The problem is that the phenolated A-ring is also common in petrochemical by-products and pesticides. Many of the offending chemicals, including organo-chlorines (examples include DDT and chlordane), have been outlawed for use in the U.S. and Canada. Unfortunately, they continue to find their way to our food products. They remain in our soils from previous use over 2 decades ago and continue to be used in some third-world countries.

The biological effect on humans by many pesticides in common use, today, is not universally agreed on. Vincent Castronova, M.D., Ph.D., noted at the 6th International Symposium on Functional Medicine (May 25, 1999), that current research suggests that 90 to 95% of all cancers are caused by environmental toxins. It is well known that these chemicals, as well as estrogens and antibiotics, are lipophilic (capable of dissolving, of being dissolved in, or of absorbing lipids—fats). They tend to accumulate in the fat of the animals we eat and, eventually, are stored in our own fat tissue. Exposure may result in either acute (short-term) or chronic (long-term) biological effects. The acute effects occur immediately after heavy exposure to pesticides and have been well documented by the scientific community. The chronic effects develop over a longer period of time and last for several years after initial exposure. The effect may be related to a long-term repeated exposure of a pesticide at a low dosage or to exposure at a higher dosage over a short to moderate period of time. Chronic health effects typically include cancer, interference with the development of the fetus and child, and disruption of the reproductive, endocrine, immune and/or central nervous systems.

Toxins and Pesticides

A real problem results from the fact that many common household products are considered pesticides. The U.S. EPA (Environmental Protection Agency) defines a pesticide as any substance or mixture of substances intended for preventing, destroying, repelling, or mitigating any pest. These pests can be insects, mice and other animals, unwanted plants (weeds), fungi, or microorganisms like bacteria and viruses. Though often misunderstood to refer only to insecticides, the term pesticide also applies to herbicides, fungicides, and various other substances used to control pests. Under United States law, a pesticide is also any substance or mixture of substances intended for use as a plant regulator, defoliant, or desiccant. In accordance with the definition by the *EPA Office of Pesticide Programs* (February 14, 1997), the following common products are considered pesticides:

- Cockroach sprays and baits
- Insect repellents for personal use.
- Rat and other rodent poisons.
- Flea and tick sprays, powders, and pet collars.
- Kitchen, laundry, and bath disinfectants and sanitizers.
- Products that kill mold and mildew.
- Some lawn and garden products, such as weed killers.
- Some swimming pool chemicals.

By their very nature, most pesticides create risk of harm to humans, animals, or the environment because they are designed to kill or otherwise adversely affect living organisms.

According to the *EPA Office of Pesticide Programs* (updated July 12, 2001), the following are not considered pesticides:

- Drugs used to control diseases of humans or animals (such as livestock and pets) are not considered pesticides; the Food and Drug Administration regulates such as drugs.
- Fertilizers, nutrients, and other substances used to promote plant survival and health are not considered plant growth regulators and, thus, are not pesticides.

· The EPA exempts biological control agents, except for certain microorganisms, from regulation. (Biological control agents include beneficial predators, such as birds or ladybugs, which eat insect pests.)
· Finally, EPA has also exempted certain other low-risk substances, such as cedar chips, garlic, and mint oil.

While these products do not officially qualify as pesticides, they are part of the estimated 87,000 plus chemicals that are commercially used today. Of these, 465 toxic and persistent chemicals are approved for use on conventional produce. Approximately 3,000 chemical compounds are regularly used in skin and beauty products. This brings the issue of endocrine disruptors (ED) to the forefront of concern, today. Endocrine disruptors are man-made synthetic chemicals and natural phytoestrogens (*plant products that behave biologically similar to natural estrogen*) that act on the endocrine systems by mimicking, blocking, and/or interfering in some manner with natural hormonal function of cells.

It's a Matter of Exposure

There are a number of issues related to chemical exposure and endocrine disruptors. While there is not total agreement within the fields of science and medicine on these theories, I believe that enough evidence exists to present them for your consideration.

The first is the matter of *synergy*. It means that the combination of more than one chemical can have the synergistic effect (think of it as 1 + 1 equaling something more than 2) of increasing the toxicity many times above that of each chemical separately. A second concern is *bioaccumulation* (the process of increased concentrations of chemicals as one species of fish or animal feeds on lesser species). The concentrations of EDs are magnified through the process of bioaccumulation up the food chain. The accumulation of EDs in the fatty tissues of animals and fish at the top of the food chain can be millions of times higher than the concentration found in the water that the chemical, first, came to rest in. This is particularly relevant to consumers with the recommendation by the government to increase fish consumption and the consequent increased exposure to mercury. The accumulation of mercury in the body can have serious effects, including elevated cholesterol, increased incident of heart attack, cancer, autoimmune diseases, and elevated blood pressure.

The FDA (Food and Drug Administration) has compiled a list of fish with their respective amounts of mercury (bad) and omega-3 fatty acids (good).

The fish and seafood with the lowest levels of mercury include:

· Shrimp
· Salmon
· Flounder or sole
· Crab
· Canned tuna
· Mahi-mahi
· Herring
· Pollack

Moderate mercury levels are found in:

·   Halibut
·   Lobster
·   Fresh tuna
·   Orange roughy
·   Red snapper.

The highest levels can be found in:

·   King mackerel
·   Shark
·   Swordfish
·   Tilefish (golden snapper).

These highest-level fish tend to be predator fish and occupy the top of the food chain. The FDA recommends that you eat no more than 7 ounces of these fish per week. My advice is to avoid them all together. When you buy fish, generally pick the smaller ones; they have not lived as long and therefore have had less exposure to toxins. According to a 2003 study published in the *Journal of the American Medical Association,* 8% of women of childbearing age have unacceptably high levels of mercury in their bodies. Women with elevated levels of mercury tend to have children with developmental delays and learning disabilities.

The third area of concern is the vulnerability of infants and children to toxicants (any poisonous agent). Children's metabolic pathways, especially in the first months after birth, are immature compared to those of adults and generally less able to detoxify these chemicals from their systems. Infants and children are growing and developing and their delicate developmental processes and immune systems are easily disrupted. The resulting dysfunction can be permanent and irreversible if: pesticides affect the cells in an infant's brain, endocrine disrupters divert the reproductive development, or the maturation of the immune system is altered. Because children have more future years of life, they will have more time in which to develop chronic disease. These diseases may be initiated as a result of early exposures to toxins and endocrine disruptors.

Significant exposure to endocrine disruptors is from plastic, which is displacing natural products at an ever-increasing pace. Of all plastics, PVC (polyvinyl chloride) probably contributes the greatest exposure to EDs. It is toxic during production, use, and when it is disposed of. PVC is made into residential and municipal water pipes, toys, food wrap, clothing, shoes, building products, such as windows, siding, roofing, flooring, and medical equipment, such as hospital blood bags, IV bags, tubing, and many other devices. Polystyrene (a plastic material) is made into food containers, foam and rigid plates, clear bakery containers, packaging materials, foam packaging, audiocassette housings, CD cases, and disposable cutlery. To be fair and balanced, a survey conducted through the State of Wisconsin Cancer Registry, revealed no conclusive relationship between plastics and increased breast cancer risk. In my opinion, the findings of this survey should be taken in context: one material's effect on one type of cancer. I would therefore recommend, when possible, be conservative in the usage of these noted materials.

Oil refining, the burning of coal and oil for energy, all auto and truck exhaust, and cigarette smoke create endocrine disruptors. The use of synthetic lawn chemicals, household cleaners, paints, solvents, waxes, and thousands of commonly used products put people into direct contact with EDs.

In reality, there are thousands of manmade synthetic products that act as endocrine disruptors. With a few exceptions, one cannot place blame for the problem on one chemical, but on the principles of bioaccumulation, synergy, and early exposures. Current regulations are being aimed at individual chemicals; in fact, the combinations are infinite and may have unpredictable effects.

Cosmetics

To me, fair friend, you can never be old,
For as you were when first your eye I eyed,
Such seems your beauty still.
—William Shakespeare

Contrary to the above lines from Shakespeare, we are in a constant quest to retain the beauty of our youth, a fight against the inevitable march of time. Such has been the battle for centuries. For seventeen centuries women used a European cosmetic, ceruse, to make their skin look fashionably pale. The main ingredient in ceruse was white lead, and its repeated use often had fatal consequences. Today, cosmetic safety falls into a category at best defined as an "inexact science." The Food and Drug Administration (FDA) oversees the Federal Food, Drug, and Cosmetic Act. This provision is, in a way, a double-edged sword. Its enactment was intended to safeguard consumer health and economic interest. At the same time, it contained language to protect a manufacturer's right to market a product free of excess government regulation. What remains today is an industry controlled, to a great extent, through self-regulation and compliance to accepted industry standards. The FDA encourages industry participation in these associations, the most well known being the Cosmetic Ingredient Review (sponsored by the Cosmetic Toiletry and Fragrance Association). Unfortunately, the FDA estimates that approximately 35% of the cosmetic manufacturing and marketing firms participate.

For our discussion on cosmetics, let's review a few basic principles. Our goal is health, not the absence of symptoms. Our health, especially hormonal balance, can be affected by what is put "on" and "in" the body. Repeated exposure to chemicals in cosmetics, whether natural or synthetic, may result in hormonal imbalance as a result of bioaccumulation and synergy.

The FDA has classified cosmetics into 13 categories:

1. Skin care (creams, lotions, powders, and sprays)
2. Fragrances
3. Eye makeup

4. Manicure products
5. Makeup other than eye (lipstick, foundation, and blush)
6. Hair conditioning preparations
7. Shampoos, permanent waves, and other hair products
8. Deodorants
9. Shaving products
10. Baby products
11. Bath oils and bubble bath
12. Mouthwashes
13. Tanning products

The FDA prohibits the use of the following products:

1. Biothionol
2. Hexachlorophene
3. Mercury compounds
4. Vinyl chloride and zirconium salts in aerosol products
5. Chloroform
6. Methyl chloride

The above noted lists those products that the FDA has "outlawed" all together. Of greater concern to you, the consumer is the effect of ingredients that are legal and in use today.

Common consumer complaints concerning cosmetic use are: first, allergic reaction to fragrances, and second, allergic reaction resulting from preservatives. Symptoms related to these allergic reactions are: headache, dizziness, rashes, skin discoloration, coughing, and vomiting. Fragrance, products that enhance the smell of a cosmetic, can be a combination of synthetic and natural ingredients. It is estimated that literally thousands of chemicals can be mixed to produce today's fragrances. Cosmetic containers may only indicate the presence of added fragrance, thus making it impossible to know the exact ingredients. The term hypoallergenic, commonly assumed to mean "will not cause allergic reaction," is a misnomer. In reality, it is the manufacturer's statement to indicate that a product is *less likely to cause* an allergic reaction or irritation than other similar products. Some cosmetic firms do clinical testing and trials, but many base their statement on the fact that they simply omit common problem-causing ingredients. A previously used test for determining adverse reactions to cosmetics was the Draize Eye Irritancy Test. Due to the fact that this procedure involved animal testing, it has fallen from popular use by many firms. Statements noting, "no animals used in testing," refer to the fact that the current product has not been tested on animals. In reality, most of the clinical information relevant to product safety is based on prior testing. Many firms base their safety statements on the fact that the ingredients are "natural." Even natural products can be the cause of reactions when used in excess or in combination with other ingredients.

Herein lies the next area of confusion: you have purchased a product from a reputable company, and then made the mistake of trying to read the ingredients list. An inclusive list of cosmetic ingredients is prohibitive in this text. I highly recommend that you download a useful tool before you make your next trip to the cosmetic counter. Dean Coleman has posted the "Cosmetic Ingredients Reference Guide & Dictionary" at www.deancoleman.com/cosmetics.htm. This guide does not indicate which ingredients are considered good or bad but merely describes them in an effort to "identify the mysterious names commonly found on labels."

Have You Tried Reading the Label?

Dean Coleman describes them as "mysterious names" and that they are! A degree in chemistry would help, but it is not necessary if you understand a few basic things about cosmetic ingredients and marketing. When reading a label, the first thing to understand is that ingredients are listed in descending order of predominance. That is, the ingredient with the greatest concentration is listed first, the second highest concentration next, and so on.

Common Cosmetic Terms

Hypoallergenic: indicates the product does not contain common allergens such as preservatives and perfumes. This is the manufacturer's statement the product is *less likely to cause* a reaction.

Allergy-tested: indicates the manufacturer has performed skin-allergy patch test. No government regulations means the tests may have been performed on only one person, or a thousand. Additionally, there is no guarantee the tests were conducted on humans.

Dermatologist-tested: the product has been "tested" by a dermatologist. But, without standards, this can mean anything from the physician merely trying the product out, or actually conducting extensive tests. Who knows?

Noncomedogenic: the product should not clog skin pores as a result of not containing heavy emollients, like mineral oil.

Nonacnegenic: the product should not inflame or irritate the oil-producing follicles (causing pimples). Generally indicates the product does not contain heavy oils.

Fragrance or Perfume-free: indicates that no natural or synthetic scents have been added to the product.

Unscented: the product should have no fragrance at all—though a masking scent may be added to achieve this quality. The added ingredient may cause a skin reaction.

Preservative Free: Manufactured without traditional preservatives. May contain some ingredient to maintain "freshness" *not expected* to cause a skin reaction.

Oil-free: the product has been manufactured without the inclusion of heavy oils. May contain additives such as dimethicone (silicone).

There are a few absolutes when purchasing cosmetics. Avoid all products that are manufactured from petroleum distillates (petrochemicals). The most common offender is mineral oil. Baby oil is a frequently used mineral oil product. An application of baby oil coats the skin, impeding its normal functions of excretion (breathing) and absorption. The oily coating leeches the vitamins and moisture from the top layers of the skin, leaving it undernourished and ultimately drier.

We are familiar with isopropyl alcohol (rubbing alcohol). Most have a bottle in the bathroom, using it to sanitize surfaces or sterilize objects. It is a solvent, a substance that helps dissolve or breakdown other substances. Isopropyl alcohol is commonly found in hair color rinses, body rubs, hand lotions, after-shave products, and fragrances. It is readily adsorbed into the skin and with excess topical applications (rubbing it on the skin) can be fatal. Inhalation or ingestion has been associated with headache, flushing, mental depression, vomiting, and coma.

Other ingredients identified as carcinogens (cancer causing) include:

- PEG: polyethylene glycol. Commonly used to make cleansers and assist in dissolving oil and grease.
- PG: propylene glycol. This is a "wetting" agent and solvent. This ingredient may be produced by mixing a vegetable glycerin and grain alcohol (and labeled natural) or as a synthetic petrochemical mixture. It is found in its highest concentration in stick deodorants. Mouthwash and toothpaste may also contain propylene glycol. PG is the active ingredient in the industrial manufacture of antifreeze. It can quickly penetrate the skin and factory workers are required by the EPA to wear protective clothing.
- Sodium Lauryl Sulfate (SLS) is a synthetic substance found in shampoos noted for it's foaming and degreasing properties. It is closely related to industrial products including car wash soaps, floor cleaners, and engine degreasers. It is a common ingredient in toothpaste, hair conditioners, and all foaming products. Common allergic reactions to SLS exposure include eye irritation, skin rashes, and hair loss. Due to its ability to penetrate the skin, questions have been raised about organ toxicity.
- DEA-diethanolamine, MEA-monoethanol-amine, TEA-triethanolamine: are compounds associated with neutralizing other compounds. An example of a product ingredient listing is Lauramide DEA. This and similar compounds have been identified as endocrine disruptors (EDs). They are commonly found in personal care products that foam, including bubble bath, shampoos, and facial cleansers. Due to their rapid skin

absorption, their repeated use has been identified as a risk, especially to children.

- Imidazolidinyl urea and diazolidinyl urea: these are two common cosmetic preservatives and are associated with the release of formaldehyde. The American Academy of Dermatology has identified both as causes of contact dermatitis (skin irritation). These may be listed under their trade names of Germall II and Germall 115.
- Methyl paraben (may also be listed as propyl, butyl, or ethyl paraben): these ingredients are used as anti-microbials and to extend shelf life of cosmetics. They have been associated with allergic reactions and skin rashes.
- Acetone is a flammable, colorless liquid used in nail polish and nail polish removers. Excess exposure to the skin and inhaling acetone can be extremely toxic.

Due to allergic and anaphylactic reactions, care should be taken when a cosmetic contains synthetic colors. The label containing the following identifies them: FD&C (or D&C) followed by a color name or number (example: FD&C Red Dye No.6). The FD&C indicates that the FDA has certified the coloring ingredient to be safe in food, drugs, and cosmetics (D&C indicates safety in drugs and cosmetics, but not food).

Some final thoughts on cosmetics: do not share and throw out old products! Sharing, especially mascara brushes, invites the transfer of germs to the eyes. The surface of the eyeball (cornea) is easily scratched, leading to possible contamination of the eye and surrounding structures. A common method of self-contamination results from scratching the eye when applying mascara while driving (it only takes one bump in the road).

Industry experts recommend discarding mascara after 3 months. Other makeup products may be kept longer but should be thrown out if there is a noticeable change in color or odor. This may indicate that the preservative in the product has degraded and will no longer protect you from bacterial growth. All makeup products should be kept away from sunlight and heat, both of which contribute to ingredient breakdown. Adding water or saliva to bring a product back to its normal consistency is never appropriate. Consistency changes are another indication of preservative breakdown. Whenever possible, you should purchase products that have airtight containers. Pump applicators, in which the bottom of the container rises as the product is expressed, keep air from degrading the ingredients. When this type of container is not available, always close the lid tightly.

Practical Application

- One way to start this clean up is to buy organic. Certified organic meats, poultry, milk and eggs are available at many major supermarkets. Organic vegetables generally require shopping at a health food store or organic farmer's market. All vegetables and fruits should be rinsed thoroughly in clean water.

-

- Drinking water should, at a minimum, be filtered.

- Do not smoke, and make every effort to avoid second-hand smoke.

- Avoid all products that contain mineral oil and other petroleum distillates. Using Baby Oil is a frequent offender for the average mother or sun worshipper. Acetone nail polish removers and other products related to artificial nails are other sources to be avoided. Utilize a company (Arbonne International) that offers a complete line of body products, soaps, cosmetics and beauty aids that are environmentally sensitive and do not add to the estrogen dominance imbalance.

- Do not use commercial lawn chemicals and pesticides. When you mow, mulch. Use plain untreated paper for weed control. There are a number of environmentally friendly products that will control pests on your flowers and vegetables.

- Use appropriate protective clothing and breathing filters when working around pesticides, petroleum products, and other toxic materials. Make sure that your work area is well ventilated.

- Do not heat food in plastic containers. Use glass or stoneware in the microwave. Do not cover dishes in the microwave with plastic wrap.

- Eat lower on the food chain.

- Eat fresh, deep-water fish. Avoid farm-raised fish that have been exposed to chemicals, including estrogens for fattening and antibiotics.

- Use fewer processed, prepackaged foods whenever possible. Prepare a week's worth of meals in advance, and freeze them. To assist with this, I recommend adding a vacuum sealer to your kitchen appliances (the FoodSaver by Tilia has been an absolute indispensable part of our food preparation).

- Avoid foods that contain hydrogenated or partially hydrogenated fats. Avoid fats and oils that smell rancid. These will result in cellular function damage.

- Understand that not all "natural" cosmetics are good for you. Become label readers for cosmetics and beauty products.

- Do not throw away the box that a cosmetic product comes in. Many times, it will be the only place that the ingredients are listed. Compare the ingredients to those you should avoid before actually using it.

- Understand "puffery" in the cosmetic industry. Puffery is the use of "gimmick" ingredients for promotion and sale. Puffery does not require scientific substantiation and often walks on the edge of making fraudulent and misleading claims.

Part Five

Prescription Estrogen
(and other hormones)

Before you ask another question, remember:
I have PMS and a gun!
—An anonymous receptionist

An Overview

Estrogen.... it seems to be everywhere in the news! Sooner or later, every woman will have to make an important decision regarding hormonal issues. That decision needs to be based on fact, not fear and confusion.

The sex hormones are primarily composed of estrogens, progesterone, and testosterone. Both female and male have these in variable amounts. All, including cortisol and DHEA, are made from circulating cholesterol.

Estrogen is a collective term for (E1) estrone, (E2) estradiol, and (E3) estriol. Estradiol is the most physiologically active in the non-pregnant and premenopausal female and is 12 times as potent as estrone. Estradiol is primarily produced in the ovaries and the adrenal cortex (outer layer). Due to its potency, estradiol plays a major role in female sexual development, menstrual function, protein synthesis, cardiovascular function, bone development, and cognitive and emotional factors. Estrogen stimulates deposition of fat tissue in subcutaneous tissue, especially the breast. After menopause, estrone becomes the main estrogen as the ovaries loose their ability to manufacture estradiol. Estrone is produced in the adrenal glands and the peripheral fat tissue. It is not unusual for obese women to have higher circulating levels of estrone. Estriol is the weakest of the estrogens, and its function is not completely clear.

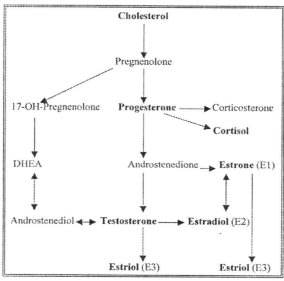

Progesterone - the body manufactures two forms: 1) progesterone and 2) 17-alpha hydroprogesterone. The former is considered the primary active progesterone as hydroprogesterone is produced in minute quantities. Progesterone is produced in the ovaries and adrenal glands in non-pregnant women. The three major functions of progesterone are: 1) the survival and development of the fetus, 2) a broad range of internal biological functions, and 3) as a precursor of other steroid hormones (see previous chart).

Testosterone plays an important role in maintaining lean body mass in the adult female. It also contributes to bone density, skin elasticity, and libido. Low testosterone levels may be related to increased risk of osteoporosis and may suggest ovarian insufficiency and/or adrenal dysfunction. Elevated levels have been noted in polycystic ovary disease, masculinization, and with increased risk of insulin resistance.

Hormones do not work in isolation. An excellent summary of this balance between estrogen and progesterone by James N. Brenner, M.A., notes:

> Each one is part of a vast complex network of other hormones and metabolic mediators. Progesterone and estrogen work essentially as a team even though their respective roles appear to be opposing. The resulting effect of their respective roles is due to their delicate balance. In breast tissue, estrogen stimulates breast duct cells to proliferate. Progesterone on the other hand inhibits this proliferation, causing maturation and differentiation, which makes them more resistant to cancerous, cells. This is true in both premenopausal and menopausal women. Breast duct cell proliferation is considered to be an early sign of the changes that lead to breast cancer. The evidence of progesterone's protectiveness isn't hard to understand. In 1981 L.D. Cowan and colleagues at John Hopkins published in the American Journal of Epidemiology their findings that women who were deficient in progesterone were 5.4 times more likely to acquire breast cancer, and 10 times more likely to develop cancer of any sort. In women with node-positive breast cancer, P.E. Mohr and coworkers found in 1996 that women with normal progesterone levels at the time of the breast cancer surgery had an 18-year survival rate which was twice that of women with low progesterone levels at the time of their surgery. This is an extremely significant finding. In March 1998 the National Cancer Institute convened a symposium on the role of estrogen as a cause of breast and prostate cancer. Dr. E.A. Cole Cavalieri of the University of Nebraska's cancer research center has discovered the metabolic steps that convert estradiol and

estrone (but not estriol) into DNA-mutating catechol estrogen quinines leading to breast cancer. Dr Jose Russo of the Fox Chase Cancer Center in Philadelphia and professor of Pathology at the University of Pennsylvania Medical School has demonstrated that human chorionic gonadotropin (HCG), a hormone released during pregnancy, prevents breast cancer by promoting maturation of breast lobules, making them less susceptible to estrogen-induced cancer. Also, in 1998 researchers B. Formby and T.S. Wiley of the Sansum Medical Research Foundation in Santa Barbara, California, showed in the annals of clinical and laboratory science that estrogen added to breast cancer cell cultures activated the oncogene (cancer-causing gene) BcL-2, whereas progesterone activated the cancer-protective gene p53. In 1996, Dr. William Hrushesky, of the Stratton VA Medical Center in Albany, New York, outlined (in the Journal of Women's Health), seven known metabolic mechanisms by which progesterone protects against breast cancer.
  —James N. Brenner, M.A., GNP-BC, and Linda Brenner
  www.faithforceonline.com

The utilization of prescription estrogen and progestin has come under increasing question. Historically, the utilization of the hormones became popular in the 70s. Unfortunately, empirical evidence on efficacy and safety trailed the widespread usage by physicians. Numerous studies of various sizes have been completed or are continuing (see "What the Studies Say"). In July 2002, a clinical trial of 16,000 women (Women's Health Initiative) was terminated early due to increased risk to those participating in it. The findings indicated that, contrary to previous reports, the combination of estrogen and progestin (a popular drug being Prempro) increased a woman's chances of blood clot, breast cancer, heart disease, and stroke. Prior to the mid 70s, women were prescribed estrogen as a stand-alone replacement following hysterectomy or to offset the symptoms of menopause. Following that time, it was found that women with an intact uterus experienced reduced uterine cancer when a progestin was added to estrogen. The National Institutes of Health estimated that 22.3 million prescriptions for Prempro were issued in 2000.

What the Studies Say

ERT: abbreviation for estrogen replacement therapy. Typically prescribed for women without their uterus.

HRT: abbreviation for hormone replacement therapy. This includes the use of estrogen and progesterone or a progestin and may or may not include testosterone supplementation.

Nurses Health Study: started in 1976 and funded by the Federal government to determine whether oral contraceptives increased the risk of breast cancer. 121,700 married nurses, age 30 to 55, answered a questionnaire every 2 years. A significant finding was that breast cancer incidence increased with each year of Estrogen Replacement Therapy usage.

Postmenopausal Estrogen/Progestin Intervention (PEPI): a randomized study of 900 women without previously known health problems. At the end of 3 years, the study found that 1) ERT, taken by itself, caused endometrial hyperplasia (a thickening of the uterine lining)—an increased risk factor for uterine cancer; 2) all types of HRT prevented this increased risk factor; 3) ERT and HRT slowed bone loss associated with osteoporosis; 4) both ERT and HRT increased breast density, making mammograms more difficult to interpret; and 5) ERT, by itself, had a positive effect on cholesterol levels—(it found that the synthetic progestin, Provera, interfered with this beneficial effect while oral micronized progesterone did not). The study was just 3 years and not considered long enough to determine the effects on breast cancer and heart disease.

Heart and Estrogen/Progestin Replacement Study (HERS): a 4-year randomized study of 2,763 women with previous heart disease (heart attack or angina). The goal was to determine whether or not hormones helped prevent the disease from worsening. In the first year of the study, women who took Premarin and Provera were more likely to have a second heart attack than women taking a placebo. The effect reversed itself by the fourth year.

Estrogen Replacement and Atherosclerosis (ERA): similar to HERS in that it followed women with preexisting heart disease. The study evaluated 309 women taking Premarin, Premarin and Provera (PremPro), or a placebo. The study confirmed the findings of both PEPI and HERS, showing a positive effect on cholesterol but no improvement in heart disease.

Women's Health Initiative: 25,000 healthy women were recruited in the largest randomized trial of the long-term effects of hormones for prevention ever attempted. In July 2002, a safety-monitoring board suddenly halted a part of the study (involving 16,608 women) because the women taking hormones had an increased risk of developing breast cancer, heart attack, stroke, pulmonary embolism, and blood clots over those taking a placebo. The participants taking Prempro had fewer bone fractures and less colon cancer, but the benefit did not outweigh the risk. This study was important in that it included women of color in numbers proportional to the American population. There was concern regarding the interpretation of data as it related to premenopausal women. The effected participants were all postmenopausal.

How This Applies To You

In understanding what to do, as a society, we must change our view of menopause. The changes associated with menopause are a natural, normal, physiological process.... menopause is not a disease.... it is not an estrogen deficiency! Menopause, as well as other menstrual functions, is a balancing act of all three major hormones. It is estimated that fewer than 20% of women will experience symptoms related to true estrogen deficiency. To properly deal with the possible risk factors associated with this balancing, it is important that a woman review her family history of breast cancer, heart disease, cardiovascular disease, osteoporosis, and ovarian/uterine cancer.

Laboratory testing for hormone levels may include LH (lutenizing hormone), FSH (follicle stimulating hormone), estrogen (estradiol), progesterone, testosterone (total and free), TSH (thyroid stimulating hormone), cortisol, and insulin (may be done in conjunction with glucose tolerance testing). There are other less common hormones that may be included for testing when your doctor suspects a pathological basis for your imbalance. I recommend that this type of testing be completed at 8 to 9 a.m. and, for menstruating women, at the same time each month in their menstrual cycle (*i.e.,* mid-cycle). Menopausal and postmenopausal women should try to coordinate testing to a time near the full moon portion of the monthly lunar cycle.

There are four periods when a woman will have to make a decision about the effects of her hormone balance. The first time is pre-menopause, a nebulous period of maybe ten years before menopause. During this time, you may experience random symptoms that affect your periods, your moods, and your life in general. Most lab hormone testing will be normal. It is during this time that the affects of estrogen dominance begin to appear (please see discussion on ESTROGEN DOMINENCE in the ENVIRONMENTAL ESTROGEN section). I direct you to Dr. John Lee, author of the *What Your Doctor May Not Tell You About...* series, who describes in depth the series of events that occur during this time. As previously noted, estrogen dominance may be related to a number of factors, including stress, environment estrogen exposure, prescription estrogen use, and numerous nutrition/dietary issues. One of the primary physiological causes of estrogen dominance is anovulatory periods. Each month a woman ovulates (releases an egg) at mid-cycle (day 14 of a 28 day period). The time of ovulation is associated with an increase of vaginal mucous, and in many women, an increased libido. Both of these factors are associated with increased probability of pregnancy. Once an egg (ovum) has been released, it leaves a small pit in the ovary termed the corpus luteum. The corpus luteum is responsible for the continued production of progesterone. It is this progesterone that is necessary to help balance the body's production of estrogen. Starting as early as the late twenties and into the thirties, a woman may stop ovulating every month (anovulatory periods). This occurrence becomes more common as a woman reaches her forties. Various environmental factors may increase the incidence of ovary dysfunction in younger women. Without ovulating each month, there are times when the body continues its production of estrogen without adequate amounts of balancing progesterone. Symptoms associated with this occurrence include: irregular periods, mid-cycle spotting, increased premenstrual symptoms, fluid retention, breast tenderness, reduced libido, depression, and irritability. Standard medical practice incorporates the use of oral birth control pills to regulate your periods during this time. Dr. Lee and other researchers believe that while this may relieve many of the symptoms, the end result is an increase in the estrogen dominance.

Linda D. presented with frustration over continuation of her health problems. For 2 years she had been complaining to her primary care physician and gynecologist that she did not feel well. She was fatigued, experienced anxiety and foggy thinking, migraine type headaches, decreased libido, hair loss on the head with increased facial hair, night sweats, and weight gain in spite of dieting. Linda D. was a "poster child" for estrogen dominance and was emotionally frustrated that her other doctors did not recognize it and treat it. I explained that the typical first-line medical approach was administration of antidepressants and oral birth control pills. She had been prescribed both, utilized them for a reasonable period, but did not like the side effects she experienced. Following physical examination and review of her last 2 years lab studies she was started on topical progesterone cream from days 12 to 26 of her menstrual cycle. Additionally, she started a stress reduction exercise to control chronic cortisol production. Review of a 10-day food diary resulted in dietary and food selection changes. She started on a consistent exercise regime. Over the next 3 months she experienced marked improvement regarding night sweats, headaches, PMS symptoms, libido, and hair growth on her head. At 5 months she continued with facial hair growth, mild anxiety, times (during the morning) of marked fatigue, no appreciable weight loss, and an alteration of the length of her monthly cycle. The progesterone-dosing schedule was changed to include an interim period of twice daily. She admitted not exercising as directed. Stress reduction exercises were reviewed along with additional advice on balancing her diet. At nine months she continues with marked improvement in all areas. She notes occasional episodes of anxiety but has been able to handle them with breathing exercises. This case is an example of the importance of having a doctor-patient partnership. Because all of Linda's symptoms did not resolve with the initial treatment plan, she may have been tempted to quit all together. The doctor was utilized as a resource to make appropriate "mid-course" corrections on her journey to improved health.

A comment on birth control pills: since the introduction of "the pill" in 1960, over 50 million American women have used some form of chemical contraception. The topic of a woman's reproductive rights is a thorny issue that elicits many strong opinions and emotions. The choice to use chemical contraception needs to be an informed decision—weighing the benefits against the risk. Birth control pills (this includes oral, topical, and implant methods of application) are not hormones—they are chemicals that interfere with a woman's normal hormone balance. They are usually a combination of synthetic estrogen and progestin. These chemicals suppress the body's normal hormone production and alter the monthly ovarian function. Because they are synthetic, the body, especially the liver, has to excrete the foreign chemicals from the body. It is important to understand that a change in one hormone system (in this case the sex hormones) has an affect on a number of the other hormonal systems. Unfortunately, you can never achieve normal hormonal balance while taking birth control pills. Birth control pills have been associated with increased blood clots (deep vein thrombosis), breast and uterine cancer, elevated blood pressure, altered cholesterol levels, and other symptoms associated with estrogen dominance. Other effective methods of birth control include barriers (condoms and diaphragms) and natural family planning. While all of these methods have their downsides (lack of spontaneity, tracking your period, etc.), they are not detrimental to your hormone balance.

The second hormonal timeframe of concern is peri-menopause. It is that period of approximately 1 year prior to menopause, which indicates ovarian function beginning to slow. Periods are irregular, and early symptoms may include mild occasional hot flashes, increased irritability, and forgetfulness. Many women note a marked change in the length of their monthly cycle. It

may lengthen or shorten by a week or more. Monthly flow ma,
and mid-period spotting is not unusual. Laboratory testing may
transitional period. Again, I encourage you to have your testing d
to 8 a.m. as possible. When repeat testing is done, do it at the san ˌ of
day as your previous test.

Menopause is associated with cessation of periods and may be
accompanied by night sweats, hot flashes, and severe mood swings. It is
during this period that many women contemplate the use of estrogen or
hormone replacement. It is important to understand that estrogen is not the
only hormone produced in the ovaries. Testosterone and DHEA (androgens),
as well as progesterone, are also synthesized in the ovaries. Altered ovarian
function affects all of these. It is important for hormonal balance that
adequate amounts of each of these hormones be synthesized. All of these
hormones are produced to a degree in various sites, including the adrenal
glands, muscles, and body fat. As hormone production decreases in the
ovaries, these other sites increase the production of the androgens by two-
fold. Androgens have both an estrogenic effect as well as being estrogen
precursors, and therefore, adequate production can offset the need for
supplemental estrogen. A decrease in DHEA and testosterone can have
marked affects on bone strength and libido. Consideration for supplementing
these two hormones should only be done under a physician's supervision.
Blood and/or saliva testing are accurate and necessary to determine the need
for and the effects of supplementation. DHEA, a testosterone precursor, is an
"over-the-counter" supplement, but I recommend physician monitoring to
assure that a normal physiological balance be obtained. Only a
pharmaceutical USP grade DHEA should be used.

The postmenopausal period (one year after your last period) generally
means no more disrupting symptoms but is generally associated with
increased bone resorption in the hip and spine. Increased vaginal dryness may
continue and be associated with decreased libido. Laboratory testing of
testosterone levels may be appropriate. Testosterone supplementation is
relatively inexpensive and a simple way to assure improved sexual relations
as well as improved bone density. Topical vaginal application of a
bioidentical estrogen may adequately alleviate vaginal dryness (both
testosterone and estrogen, are prescription, and the use of these needs to be
discussed with your medical doctor). Regular intercourse also improves the
body's natural lubrication. Utilizing a topical progesterone (a precursor for
estrogen) will assist in maintaining a proper estrogen-progesterone balance.
In my opinion, the only appropriate use of hormone replacement therapy
(HRT) is when indicated by a deficiency on laboratory testing or when
symptoms disrupt normal life. Prior to initiation of hormone replacement in

the perimenopausal and menopausal woman, lab testing should include evaluation of estrogen, progesterone, testosterone, and DHEA levels. When it is necessary to utilize estrogen (ERT) or estrogen-progesterone (HRT), I recommend that you request your medical doctor to prescribe a bioidentical formulation. The most common synthetic hormones prescribed are Premarin (ERT) and PremPro (HRT). Bioidentical hormones are plant based. Because of this, they cannot be patented and have gained little interest from large pharmaceutical companies that depend on the patented nature of their drugs for continuing profits. Recently, Wyeth, the manufacturer of Premarin and PremPro, has attempted to overcome the negative publicity associated with their products by introducing a lower dose version. There are currently only three (3) strengths of these synthetic hormones. The benefit of compounded bioidentical hormones is that they can be formulated to meet the specific dosage needs of the individual patient.

When hormone replacement is initiated in the postmenopausal women, a few additional tests are necessary to assure safety. Bleeding after menopause is generally associated with uterine cancer. A woman who has a uterus will be prescribed a combination of estrogen and progesterone, and bleeding similar to a period may start. To be totally sure that this bleeding is benign, I recommend that you have: 1) a pelvic ultrasound, and 2) an endometrial biopsy completed prior to or shortly after starting HRT. These two tests will assist in determining the health of the uterine tissue.

Progesterone is not commonly prescribed in association with estrogen for post-surgical menopause when the uterus has been removed. John Lee, MD, states that this will add to estrogen dominance and numerous additional symptoms. Use of supplemental topical progesterone may be adequate to offset these symptoms. (I encourage menopausal women to read *What Your Doctor May Not Tell You About Menopause* by John Lee, M.D.)

There are numerous options to address the symptoms of hot flashes, vaginal dryness, mood swings, and the issue of osteoporosis.

HOT FLASHES—increase phytoestrogens (plant based estrogenic food) in your diet. These do not stimulate estrogen production but act in a similar, less intense manner on estrogen cell receptors. There is no evidence that they promote abnormal breast and uterine tissue growth. These include soy products (soy milk/yogurt, soy nuts, tofu, defatted soy protein—used in moderation), golden flax seed (finely ground!). Black Cohosh has been used successfully either alone or in combination with topical progesterone.

Menopausal symptoms (just like PMS, irregular menses, etc.) may not be just from a deficiency of estrogen production. Similar symptoms may indicate estrogen dominance when progesterone synthesis is low, and the balance of the two hormones is off. When progesterone is low, utilizing Vitex (prior to total ovarian cessation) or topical/vaginal suppository progesterone cream is extremely beneficial. It is appropriate to have the levels of hormones measured using either blood or saliva test to assist in establishing an adequate protocol of care.

VAGINAL DRYNESS—vaginal creams and lubricants can help maintain a normal sex life. Progesterone, topically applied, may help maintain tissue integrity. Prescription medications include Vagifem and Estring. If a prescription medication is necessary, I recommend consideration of bioidentical estriol cream applied to the vaginal tissue. Estriol is believed not to cause abnormal cell proliferation.

MOOD SWINGS—a diet that balances insulin and blood sugar levels has a marked affect on energy levels and mood. Maintaining healthy sleeping habits and exercise also help. Omega-3 fatty acids, tryptophan rich foods (almonds, cottage cheese, oatmeal, peanut butter, peanuts, soy foods, tuna, and turkey) help balance serotonin levels. When administering St John's Wort and 5-HTP, it is recommended that a physician monitor its use. Evaluation of glucose, insulin, cortisol, and thyroid levels is appropriate when mood swings are associated with marked periods of fatigue. Cyclic periods of fatigue in both the a.m. (mid-morning) and p.m. (mid-afternoon) may be associated with fluctuating blood sugar levels. This will be further discussed in the section on nutrition. Late p.m. fatigue may indicate an alteration of the normal daily rhythms of cortisol production. Adequate sleep in a darkened environment is necessary for melatonin (a hormone produced in the pineal gland of the brain when it becomes dark) to control the production of cortisol in the adrenal glands. Elevated a.m. cortisol indicates that the body is out of synch with the normal daily time clock by 8-12 hours. Typically, these individuals are under extreme stress and become energized as the evening to late night hours approach. Sleep dysfunction is common with a feeling of never being refreshed on arising in the morning. If you have traveled internationally or across multiple time zones, you have probably experienced this sensation—"jet lag." Individuals with elevated a.m. cortisol are basically stuck in a constant state of jet lag. Over-the-counter melatonin has been approved by the FDA for correction of jet lag and can be used to "reset" the body clock associated with elevated a.m. cortisol. To correct altered a.m. cortisol:

Utilize a pharmaceutical grade melatonin. Plan on going to bed between 10 and 11 p.m.. Prior to retiring take 1 mg of melatonin. Do not leave on any lights, including nightlights in the bathroom. Upon arising between 6-8 a.m. stare "blankly" into a small flashlight for 30 seconds. (Do not look directly into the light but focus on an object across the room while gazing into the light.) This bright light causes the body to shut off the production of melatonin and start the rise of cortisol. In essence the body shuts down the nightly repair processes associated with sleep and starts the active productive phase.

It has been estimated that a significant percentage of Americans are sleep deprived. Immeasurable dollars, work production, and lives (accidents) are lost as the result of the consequences related to sleep deprivation.

OSTEOPOROSIS—estrogen has a protective affect on bone, but only while it is being taken. Once estrogen use is terminated, the body returns to its normal level of bone turnover. It is important for perimenopausal women to have a base line DEXA scan completed. A bone resorption urine test is an easy way to monitor the success of a program of care. The current medications utilized for osteoporosis in addition to estrogen are Fosamax and Actonel. Both of these medications can be taken one time per week, but a significant percentage (estimated at 30-50%) of the women that start will discontinue within one year as a result of side effects or cost issues. The main side effect is gastric reflux and ulceration. An alternative medication, Reloxifene (Evista) prevents fractures without the increased breast cancer risk. Unfortunately, many women experience increased hot flashes and blood clots on this medication. There is also concern that it may increase cognitive dysfunction since it is classified as a SERM (select estrogen receptor modulator) and therefore blocks brain cells from the protective benefits of the estrogen still being produced in the other tissues (other than the ovaries). Nonprescription ipriflavone, a phytoestrogen derivative, has been shown to be efficacious and safe for the treatment of osteoporosis. Ipriflavone must be taken 3 times per day and therefore has a low level of compliance. All methods noted should be combined with an appropriate diet including supplemental calcium and/or vitamin D, weight bearing exercise, insulin balance (decreases pro-inflammatory cascades), and avoidance of excess alcohol, caffeine, and smoking. Progesterone and testosterone, both have positive affect on bone building (osteoblast) and, therefore, should be evaluated with lab testing and supplemented as needed.

Practical Application

·   Supplement with Omega-3 (pharmaceutical grade fish oil) and GLA (Evening Primrose or Borage Oil).

·   Exercise for 20-45 minutes 3-5 days per week. This must be weight bearing—walking, biking, etc. Utilize hand weights 2 times per week for strength training.

·   Practice a stress reduction exercise daily.

·   Eat an anti-inflammatory type diet (see under nutrition section). Start a diet with increased phytoestrogens (soy, flax).

·   When appropriate, supplement with hormone replacement.

·   For hot flashes and night sweats, try Black Cohosh—160 mg twice per day.

·   For sleep dysfunction, try melatonin (1 mg) or inositol (500 mg) before retiring at night.

·   Balance insulin levels and blood glucose levels by eating protein at every meal; avoid excess red meat, and never go more than 4-5 hours without eating.

Premenopause—discuss your symptoms with a doctor who understands your concerns—you are not going crazy. This is the time to pay attention to the importance of stress reduction, the affects of xenoestrogens/xenobiotics (those chemicals and hormones you get from foods and the environment), and nutritional matters. Utilizing topical progesterone in association with life style changes may minimize the effects if the symptoms are related to estrogen dominance.

If you are not under a doctor's supervision and want to try a topical progesterone for a short period, do the following:

- Use a brand that has the USP or "GMP Certified" seal. This indicates that it is produced under specific guidelines.
- The container should be a "pump" type that seals the contents from the outside air (this oxidizes and weakens the progesterone).
- Apply ¼ teaspoon (1 pump) each p.m. starting on the 12th day of your period (consider day 1 as the first day that you bleed). Continue application through day 26 (considering that your cycle is normally 28 days). If your normal cycle is over 28 days, try stopping the progesterone on day 26, anyway, to see if your cycle will regulate to 28 days. When you stop on the 26th day, your period should start 2 days later. It is the withdrawal of progesterone that starts the sloughing off process in the uterus. If your symptoms have not improved in 3 months or if you experience marked breakthrough bleeding, discuss your symptoms with a physician that understands the use of progesterone supplementation. Application of the cream should be on skin that generally does not get exposure to sun. I recommend the inner arms and chest/breast area. I do not recommend application to the lower abdomen or buttock areas. Do not apply to the same area two days in a row. Start on the inside of one arm; and the next day, apply to the chest on the same side. The third day, apply the cream on the opposite chest area; the fourth day will be the inside of the opposite arm. The easiest way to remember is to start on the same side as you write with. Right handed, start with the right arm, followed by the right chest, etc. Using body lotions that contain mineral oil will slow or prevent the absorption of progesterone when applied to the skin.

Perimenopause—you may wish to have your hormone levels checked. Unless clearly indicated by these lab tests, initially attempt to treat symptoms with diet and lifestyle changes. When indicated, use supplements which are produced in GMP/USP certified labs. You generally cannot buy these in health food stores and may have to find a physician knowledgeable in their use. If you consider purchasing over-the-counter supplements, you can evaluate the level of compliance to advertised contents at www.consumerlabs.com.

Menopause—use estrogen (ERT) or estrogen—progesterone (HRT) when the benefits outweigh the risk and are medically indicated. Review your family history regarding health risk. If you decide to use ERT/HRT, consider "bioidentical" estrogen (Tri-Est), progesterone, and/or testosterone. These are prescription and must be prepared at a "compounding" pharmacy. These compounds, made from a plant base, have not had long-term studies and may have some of the same side effects as synthetic hormones. Currently, they appear to be tolerated better without the adverse effects of their synthetic counterparts. Try to use ERT/HRT short term (1 year), reevaluate your needs, and then try diet and supplements. Try supplements under your doctor's supervision. Supplements generally take 2 to 3 months to be effective - so be patient. Using topical progesterone may be beneficial used in combination with lifestyle changes. If your period has ceased, apply the progesterone cream nightly, starting on the first day of the month. Similar to the prior instructions (see Pre-menopause section), start with the same arm as the hand you write with. If you are right handed, start with the right inner arm, then the right chest region, etc. Remember not to apply the cream to the same area two days in a row. Continue through calendar day 25; then, discontinue for 5 or 6 days. This allows your progesterone cellular receptors a few days to rest, similar to their normal actions when you were having a menstrual cycle.

Post-menopause—exercise (including light resistant weights!!), the same diet as noted above, and follow-up with yearly mammograms, DEXA scans, and bone resorption urine test when indicated. Accelerated bone loss is now the main concern. This is where you will see the results of the choices you made 10, 20, or 30 years ago.

Again, I remind you of the goal of this program: to regain health through effective lifestyle changes. Unfortunately, as a result of age, degeneration, and prior choices, the body may not be able to correct hormonal imbalances without the use of supplementation. I cannot emphasize enough my distain for the "one size fits all" method of prescribing hormones. Yes, it takes an investment of time and money to get it right, but remember this is your body, not your car! While you can restore the body, you cannot totally trade it in on a "new" model. Find a doctor who will work as your health partner. When laboratory blood and/or saliva testing indicates the need for supplementation, use bioidentical hormones.

Part Six

Nutrition

I'm sick to death of pouring one-calorie soft drinks over my ice cream, using imitation mayonnaise in my potato salad, and ruining a perfectly good gravy sandwich by pouring it between two slices of diet bread. I come from a home where gravy is a beverage. I have dieted continuously for the last two decades and have lost a total of 758 pounds. By all calculations, I should be hanging from a charm bracelet. I walked by a hall mirror the other day and sucked in my stomach. Nothing moved!
—Erma Bombeck, *At Wits End*

An Overview

Walk into any bookstore, and you will be overwhelmed with the choices of books about dieting, cooking, and other topics related to what we eat. First, let me inform you that this section is NOT about dieting for the sake of weight loss. In keeping with our goal and definition of *health*, what follows will be more of a "guide" to making good lifestyle choices.

I have been a proponent of the balanced diet approach for over a decade. When you see those words, it generally refers to a nutritional approach with a balance of carbohydrates (40%), protein (30%), and fat (30%). This is the basis of the Zone Diet promoted by Barry Sears, PhD. For all intents and purpose, it is the foundation of *The South Beach Diet* by Arthur Agatston, M.D. Even the Atkins diet, after starting off on a primarily a high protein diet, reverts to a "balanced" maintenance program (for additional information see *Atkins for Life* by Robert Atkins, M.D.)

Dr. Barry Sears has a good explanation of the balanced diet on his websites (www.zoneperfect.com and www.drsears.com). Along with an excellent history of how the food pyramid has led to our current obesity problems, he has numerous resources for improving the diet.

What follows is an excerpt from Dr. Sear's text:

> Mother Nature has designed your digestive system to operate correctly when eating just two food groups: (1) lean protein, and (2) natural carbohydrates like fruits and fiber-rich vegetables.
>
> What about grains? Well, 8000 thousand years ago, there were no grains, bread or pasta. Agriculture is a very recent invention, by evolutionary standards! Evolutionarily speaking our genes still operate like we were hunter/gatherers, but we do not actually live that way. We regularly eat large quantities of dense, highly processed carbohydrates such as grains and grain-based products like pasta. These programs are designed to feed our actual genetic makeup—to give us the fuel we need, when we need it.
>
> It is not surprising that many people are caught in perpetual cycles of weight gain and weight loss. Over the past 20 years government health agencies and commercial interest have been

responsible for misinformation that has made us fat-phobic. During this time the U.S. population (as well as other countries that eat a western diet) has experienced a consistent increase in excess body fat. In November 1998, the U.S. Surgeon General declared an epidemic of obesity in America.

The problem starts with the FOOD PYRAMID. These recommendations came out in the late 60's in response to the rising epidemic of heart disease. Ever since, it has been the poster child of the high carbohydrate, low fat diet. What most people do not realize is that the medical establishment did not design this pyramid. It was designed by the U.S. Agricultural Department. The current "healthy diet" consist of about 65% carbohydrates, 15% fat, and 20% protein. We have been instructed to eat almost 11 servings a day of breads, cereal, rice, and pasta. These products are basically all refined carbohydrates. On the next level are the fruits, vegetables, meat and fish. Fats and oils are relegated to the smallest area at the top, because they are the enemy. The American Heart Association decided that the American public should eat less saturated fat in order to reduce heart disease (that's good). The government assumed we were not smart enough to just cut out saturated fat, so it urged us to cut out all fat (that's bad). Carbohydrates took up the vacuum formed by cutting out fats. When the Food Pyramid diet was created in the 60's, approximately 25% of the population was labeled as obese. Today that number is over 50%.

The Truth About Fat

We all tend to be fat phobic but, in fact, fat is an important part of a healthy diet. Dietary fat serves two purposes. First, it significantly slows your body's absorption of the meal you just ate. Second, fat signals you brain when to stop eating (it lets you know when you are satisfied. That is why you can eat a whole bag of non-fat cookies or chips and not feel satisfied). All fats are not created equal and the types of fat you eat play a critical role in your overall health. The best kind of fat is mono-unsaturated, the kind found in olive oil. Next are the omega-3 (flax seed and certain fish) and omega-6 (nuts and oils) fats. Eating fat in the proper proportions DOES NOT make you fat. To understand how people get fat let's look at the cattle and hog industry. To fatten their livestock they do not put out tubs of ice cream and butter. It is done by restricting the livestock's activity (not letting them roam freely—sounds a lot like a "couch" potato!) and feed them large amounts of complex carbohydrates, in the form grains.

Eating carbohydrates stimulates insulin production from the pancreas. Insulin turns the excess carbohydrates into fat. Dietary fat, on the other hand, does not stimulate insulin secretion. By eating the proper type and ratio of low-density carbohydrates, dietary fat, and protein, you can control your insulin production. Maintaining your insulin level within a therapeutic zone makes it possible to burn excess body fat and enjoy increased energy, improved mental focus, and increased vitality.

—Barry Sears, Ph.D.

www.zoneperfect.com, (2002)

While we are discussing dieting, let me say that in general I am not in favor of "diet" programs. My belief, like that of Diane Schwarzbein, MD, is that "you get healthy to lose weight, not lose weight to get healthy." If I had to endorse a book that people with weight issues would benefit from, I would pick Dr. Phil McGraw's recent book, *The Ultimate Weight Solution.* The reason I find this book a good approach is that it addresses the many issues that go into weight problems and not just food choices and portion control. I also highly recommend *The South Beach Diet* by Dr. Arthur Agatston, and *Entering the Zone* by Dr. Barry Sears; both are excellent texts, which include recipes to assist in implementing dietary changes. For those who ascribe to the Adkins approach, it is imperative that you read *Adkins for Life.* This final Adkins text describes a four-step process of introducing carbohydrates back into the diet: the last step is essentially an endorsement of the "balanced" diet approach.

Basic Principles

·   Nutrition is NOT the same as dieting.
·   Nutrition includes all the things that we put "on" and "in" our bodies.
·   The effect of nutrition is to fuel and/or alter the body's metabolism.
·   Metabolic processes either build-up or teardown the body's structural, neurological, and chemical/hormonal substances.
·   The ideal diet is one that is customized to the biochemical identity of each person, taking into account, food, allergens, and chemical allergens.

Understanding the Label

What follows is a typical nutritional food label. This particular one is from a Zone Bar. Afterward, I will discuss the sections and how best to understand the importance of each in an optimal nutritional plan:

Sample Food Label

Serving Size—1 bar

Servings	1
Calories	210
Fat Cal	60
Total Fat	7g
Sat Fat	3g
Cholesterol	0mg
Sodium	250mg
Potassium	10mg
Total Carb	22g
Dietary Fiber	0g
Sugars	13g
Protein	16g

Following the basic nutritional information is the "fine" print, including the % RDA (percent of the Recommended Daily Allowance) of other vitamins and minerals included. After that, will be the ingredients (in descending order) used in the manufacture the food product.

Serving Size

This is the number one offender for the average American. The front of the box or package may say "low-fat, low-carb!" and, in fact, each serving may actually be lower in each. The problem is that the package may include 4 servings, and when you eat more than the recommended serving, you have proportionally increased the total calories. Even with multiple servings, either the fat or carbohydrates may be in an acceptable range, but total calories are sure to be in excess. The FDA is considering a requirement to have manufacturers list the calories, fat, and other nutrients for the entire package, not just the per serving numbers.

Calorie

Definition: A unit of heat content or energy. The amount of heat necessary to raise 1 gram of water from 14.5–15.5°C.

A recent study noted that the total daily calories consumed by an American female have increased by approximately 25% over the last few decades. Today, an average female is taking in about 1900 calories per day, compared with the previously noted level of 1500 calories. Combine that with a sedentary lifestyle, a lack of fiber and antioxidants in the foodstuffs, and constant environmental toxin exposure, and you have a healthcare disaster in the making. The recommended level of daily calories for the average female is 1200-1500 per day depending upon the level of physical activity. Each gram of carbohydrate and protein equates to 4 calories. Each fat gram equates to 9 calories.

Fat Calories

As noted above, a gram of consumed fat counts for over twice the calories as carbohydrates and protein. In a balanced diet it is recommended that approximately 25-30% of your total daily calories be from good fats.

Total Fat

You need fat in your body to maintain health, build and repair cell wall membranes, and act as a precursor for hormones. That's the good news. The bad news is that all fats are not created equal. The "good" fats include monounsaturated, omega-6, and omega-3's. An acceptable fat is that listed as polyunsaturated. Polyunsaturated fats are found in soy, corn, safflower, and other vegetable oils. The "bad" fats are hydrogenated, trans fats, and saturated fats. Even within the good fat category, there is a balance, which needs to be appreciated, and efforts made to maintain that balance.

Included in the good fats are (monounsaturated) olive oil and canola oil, (omega-6) whole grains and legumes, nuts and seeds, and (omega-3) fish, flax seed and various nuts including black walnuts. The Food and Drug Administration has compiled a list of fish and their respective amounts of omega-3 fatty acids. Fish with low mercury levels and the highest levels of omega-3's include wild salmon and herring. Oysters are also included in this group. Canned tuna is considered low in mercury with a moderate level of omega-3's. Fresh and frozen tuna has a higher level of omega-3's but also a higher level of mercury.

Hydrogenated/trans fats are those that have been processed to increase the shelf life of the products they are in. These are associated with the frying of fast-food fare. Trans fats are "damaged" fats, and as such have been associated with increased risk of heart disease. In 2003, the FDA issued a ruling requiring food manufacturers to list the amount of trans fats. Unfortunately, the ruling does not take effect until 2006. This is sad in light of the estimate by the FDA that this will result in $1.8 billion per year savings in medical cost associated with chronic disease. Saturated fats are primarily associated with full fat dairy products, red meat and pork, the skin of chicken, coconut oil, and butter. Saturated fats give food flavor and are necessary for cell membrane formation but should be used in moderation especially if you have high blood sugar.

A general rule when shopping is to avoid polyunsaturated fats and oils (RULE OF THUMB # 1 - if you cannot understand the words on the label to describe the ingredients—DON'T BUY IT!). Avoid the hydrogenated and trans fats by not eating commercially fried foods, including chips, cookies, etc. (RULE OF THUMB # 2—if you leave it on the counter overnight, and it does not go bad/rancid—DON'T EAT IT!) Things that have a long shelf life have been chemically altered to slow the breakdown of the fats. When fat does spoil, it forms free radicals that cause additional cellular damage. Use butter in place of margarine. Make all salad dressings with olive oil and cook with canola oil. Once you have opened oils keep them, butter and dairy products, in the back of the refrigerator—not on the door where the temperature is constantly going up and down. Eat more fish or supplement with omega-3's, flax seed (ground), and nuts (almonds, pecans or walnuts) for snacks (in combination with fruits and berries).

Once you have the idea of which fats to eat, it is important to understand how to "balance" the fats in your diet. While the omega-6's are good, the standard American diet is tipped too heavily in their favor. Grains, flour, cereals, corn, and seeds are rich in linoleic acid, which is a precursor for prostaglandins (PGE2)—an inflammatory substance. An omega-6 rich diet, in association with elevated levels of insulin and estrogen, causes an acidic, pro-inflammatory environment to exist. The goal is to balance this with appropriate levels of omega-3's. If you do not eat fish 1 or 2 times per week, supplement daily with 1 to 2 grams of omega-3 oils. If you have existing arthritis, fibromyalgia, lupus, or other autoimmune conditions, you may need from 3 to 8 grams per day. If you are on blood thinning medication or prone to hemorrhage, you must use caution and gradually increase your daily consumption of fish oil. Current research has noted the importance of omega-3's in association with improvement of cardiovascular heart disease and inflammatory bowel syndromes.

Saturated Fat

Saturated fats are primarily associated with full fat dairy products, red meat and pork, chicken skin, coconut oil, and butter. Saturated fats give food flavor and should be used in moderation. The saturated fats in processed foods are of a poor quality and are to be avoided. One of the primary jobs of fat is to help the body know when to stop eating. The sensation of being full is called satiety. Upon ingesting fat, the body secretes cholecystokinin (CCK). This causes the gall bladder to release bile into the gastrointestinal system to assist in the breakdown and absorption of fat. Excess CCK production, as a result of too much fat in the diet will cause a feeling of nausea. Learning to listen to your body is important in finding the proper dietary balance. Fat is a major structural component of cell membranes (walls) and myelin sheaths (the covering around nerve cells—much like insulation around an electrical cord). If there is not adequate good fat intake, the integrity of these structures is compromised.

Cholesterol

Definition: the most abundant steroid in animal tissues, especially in bile and gallstones, and present in food, especially food rich in animal fats; circulates in the plasma joined to proteins of various densities, and plays an important role in the formation of the (lipid) fat deposits in the inner lining of arteries.

Cholesterol is essential in the formation of all of the steroid and sex hormones. The liver produces a certain amount of cholesterol daily. Additional dietary sources of cholesterol are needed for proper hormone synthesis. Generally, foods found in nature (eggs, nuts, etc.) that contain cholesterol are associated with lecithin, a compound that assists in proper utilization of the cholesterol. Processed foods containing large amounts of cholesterol should be avoided.

Sodium and Potassium

Sodium in foods is generally found in the form of salt. The Institute of Health estimates that ¾ of sodium intake comes hidden in processed and restaurant food. Used as a seasoning, high amounts can affect cellular function. Because of its water binding properties, care should be taken for patients experiencing fluid retention and elevated blood pressure. Recent research reveals that Americans get twice the amount of sodium needed but not enough potassium. This imbalance is related to hypertension. Approximately ⅓ of Americans has high blood pressure or is pre-hypertensive. Interestingly, low blood sodium levels have been found in patients with fibromyalgia. Decreased levels can be associated with lower blood pressure and dizziness when quickly changing positions (from seated to standing). New federal guidelines recommend that Americans below 50 years of age consume no more than 1500 mg of sodium per day. Additional recommendations include limiting intake to 1300 mg per day for those over 50 and 1200 mg per day for individuals over 70. On the other hand, potassium helps lower blood pressure and reduces the risk of kidney stones and bone loss. Good sources of potassium include: spinach, cantaloupe, and bananas, and other fruits and vegetables.

Carbohydrates

Definition: The group includes compounds with relatively small molecules, such as the simple sugars (monosaccharides, disaccharides, etc.), as well as macromolecular (larger) substances, such as starch, glycogen, and cellulose.

Carbohydrates are the first line of fuel that the cells need for energy. Simply put, most foodstuffs have to be reduced to a sugar in order to be utilized by the cellular furnaces, the mitochondria. Generally, carbohydrates are referred to as 1) simple and 2) complex (including starches). From the standpoint of good nutrition, it is recommended that the majority of carbohydrates consumed be in the complex form. Complex carbohydrates are longer chains of sugar molecules tied together. When eaten, they take a longer time to digest. The effect that the digestion of carbs has on the production (how quick and the amount produced) of insulin is termed a food's glycemic index. Insulin is produced in the pancreas and is needed to assist sugar cross the cell membrane (outer shell) on its trip to the mitochondria (the cells energy factories).

Certain starches cause a quicker response of insulin than pure sugar. The goal is to consume the lower glycemic index carbohydrates. In addition to a glycemic index is the affect of "glycemic load." The glycemic load is basically the glycemic index multiplied by a carbohydrate's density. An example: certain beans have a relatively low glycemic index, but the fact is they are rather compact in structure; broccoli also has a low glycemic index but is a much less dense vegetable, having a higher water content. While both have low glycemic indexes, the broccoli has a much lower glycemic load than the beans. Eating a ½ cup serving of broccoli causes a lower insulin response than ½ of rice. An excellent reference for knowing which foods fall into each category can be found at www.zoneperfect.com. Dr. Sears groups the foods as "favorable," "less favorable," and "avoid." I recommend that you copy or download the list and take it to the grocery store with.

As insulin is secreted into the blood stream, it causes the level of blood glucose (sugar) to rise or fall. The goal is to eat in a manner that keeps the blood glucose level stable, without peaks and valleys. Hypoglycemia is low blood sugar and is usually associated with a feeling of tiredness and a craving for sugar type foods. Hyperglycemia is high blood sugar and is associated with Metabolic Syndrome (Syndrome X) and adult onset diabetes (Type II).

A typical pattern for those experiencing blood sugar problems is: approximately 1½-2 hours after eating a high carbohydrate meal, they have a valley of fatigue and hunger. Think about why break time at work is mid-morning and mid-afternoon, a few hours after eating.

Syndrome X (also referred to as Metabolic Syndrome or Insulin Resistance Syndrome) is characterized by elevated insulin and blood sugar. Fasting blood glucose above 110 on a routine blood panel should be followed with testing for elevated fasting insulin levels. Technically, Metabolic Syndrome is diagnosed when 3 of the 5 following characteristics are found in an individual: abdominal obesity, a low HDL (cholesterol) to LDL ratio, elevated triglycerides, elevated blood pressure, and insulin resistance. With insulin resistance, the cell receptors for glucose become dulled to the affect of insulin. A gradual increase in the amount of insulin needed for glucose to enter the cell causes the pancreas to continue to secrete more and more. It is estimated that approximately 25% of Americans are insulin resistant with another 25% on the border.

Normal Glucose-Insulin Response

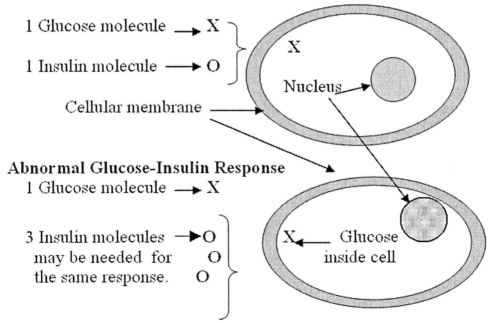

1 Glucose molecule ⟶ X

1 Insulin molecule ⟶ O

Cellular membrane ⟶

X

Nucleus ⟶

Abnormal Glucose-Insulin Response

1 Glucose molecule ⟶ X

3 Insulin molecules ⟶ O
may be needed for   O
the same response.   O

X ⟵ Glucose
inside cell

Elevated blood glucose is a major contributor for increased cholesterol. It is erroneously believed that fat causes increased blood lipids/cholesterol. In reality, a diet rich in "good" fats and low in simple carbohydrates will decrease the total cholesterol levels. When sugars enter the gut, they are transported to the liver for processing. They are stored as glycogen, formed as triglycerides, or passed on as available sugar for the cells. The breakdown of large amounts of triglycerides results in elevated LDL cholesterol (bad cholesterol). This elevation of cholesterol, in association with a pro-inflammatory circulatory system, is the major cause for the increased heart disease in America today. In spite of greatly reduced total cholesterol numbers as a result of statin type medications, Americans continue to die at an alarming rate as a result of cardiovascular disease. It needs to be mentioned, at this point, that heart disease in women and men is a different animal. While men experience a build up of plaque in the arteries, women have far less arterial blockage. Think about the last time you knew of a woman having bypass surgery. While it happens, it is rare compared to their male counterparts. Women, on the other hand, experience occlusion of the heart vessels as a result of arterial spasm. This phenomenon (occlusion related to spasm) demonstrates the importance of controlling excess cortisol production and improving the body's inflammatory status.

The typical diet in America is primarily made up of carbohydrates of poor quality. With the current craze surrounding the "low carb diet," certain facts must not be overlooked. High protein diets that are maintained over extended periods may result in potentially serious side effects. This includes increased rate of bone loss and kidney damage. While this type of diet (Atkins) results in initial weight loss and decreased cholesterol levels, recent studies indicate a loss of these benefits at approximately 1 year. Following the recommendations of the Atkins Foundation will result in the re-introduction of good carbohydrates. The final Atkins "maintenance" diet is similar to the recommendations made in this text.

Carbohydrates are a necessary part of cellular energy production and metabolism. In a study of 600 participants at MIT, Judith Wurtman, Ph.D., director of the Program in Women's Health, found a relationship between low carb diets and reduced serotonin levels. Serotonin is the neurotransmitter found in the brain that moderates mood. Decreased levels result in depression and fatigue. An intake of 130 grams of carbohydrates (520 calories) is the minimum recommended in order to maintain proper brain function.

Dietary Fiber

There are two forms of fiber: soluble and insoluble. Soluble fiber, in the intestines, turns to a gel-like substance that slows digestion and increases satiety (the feeling of being full). Insoluble fiber is not digested and, as such, attracts water to it to aid in bowel movement. Fiber will not cause insulin levels to rise. To determine insulin-stimulating grams of carbohydrates, subtract the grams of fiber on the label from the total carbohydrates listed. An excellent source for fiber is in whole grain products, ground golden flax seed, and non-starchy cruciferous vegetables (broccoli, cauliflower, kale and mustard greens). When choosing similar foods, make an effort to eat those with higher fiber contents. Generally, higher fiber foods are lower in calories. A daily goal of 25 grams of fiber is recommended.

Fiber is an important element that assists with proper elimination of feces and various substances, including cholesterol. When the body is in balance, the cells utilize the building block materials as needed and process the unused and other noxious substances out of the body. Proper bowel function is necessary to rid the body of waste materials. Good bowel habits are 1-2 bowel movements per day. Hydration, in the form of fluid consumption, is associated with proper fiber function. Recommendations for the amount of water per day vary but the rule of 8 glasses (8 oz) is generally adequate. This will be affected by one's activity level. A better method for determining total hydration is: 1½ ounces of fluid per kilogram of body weight (1 kilogram equals 2.2 pounds). This would include all liquids, including coffee and tea. Remember to drink on a consistent basis throughout the day and not just when you realize you are thirsty. If you get to that point, your body is becoming dehydrated. This is especially true during the winter, when you are not aware of sweating, and when at high altitude (including flying!)

Sugars

Most sugars in manufactured foods are refined and can be found under a number of names. These include: sucrose, fructose, maltose, dextrose, maltodextrin, polydextrose, corn syrup, and molasses. Various forms of alcohols are also used as sweeteners. High levels of sugar consumption, in addition to being calorie laden, lead to increased acidity in the blood stream and cells. The fluid inside the cell is termed cytoplasm—it has descriptively been called cellular soup. It is where the other cellular structures reside. The cytoplasm, much like the blood, urine, and saliva has an acid—base (pH) balance. An acidic environment is pro-inflammatory and leads to increased free radical production (cellular damage). The ingestion of sugar has to be dealt with by the production of insulin, and excess insulin production accelerates the disease processes. Excess blood sugar, not needed for immediate cell energy, is converted to, and stored as, fat.

The U.S. Department of Agriculture reports that in 1998 Americans on average were consuming 20 teaspoons of added sweeteners daily. This is 50% more than just 2 decades earlier. This does not count the sugar taken in through natural means in fruits and milk. The U.S.D.A. noted that in 1999 American's averaged 158 pounds of sugar per person. Robert Murray, Director of the Center for Nutrition and Wellness at the Children's Hospital in Columbus, Ohio, notes that teenage boys derive 9% of their daily calories from sugars in soda. Girls get 8% percent from sodas. Data from the University of Minnesota noted that children, aged 6 to 12, who consumed 9 ounces or more of soft drinks daily, ingested 200 calories per day more than those children who did not. A two-year study at Children's Hospital Boston indicated the risk of obesity in children rose 60% per serving of sugar-sweetened drinks ingested. The FDA has been asked by consumer groups to add "total added sugars" to the nutrition label. This would result in, as example, a notice that 9 teaspoons of sugar are added to the average can of soda. Unfortunately, merely changing to sugar free drinks will not remedy the problem. There is current concern over the long-term effects of popular sugar substitutes, including Sweet-N-Low, Equal, and Splenda. While it requires some experimentation and an acquired taste, I recommend trying Stevia in place of table sugar.

A long-term study at Loma Linda University School of Medicine revealed that a 50-gram per day intake of dietary sugar resulted in a decrease of immune function. Phagocyte (a cell possessing the property of ingesting bacteria, foreign particles, and other cells) activity was reduced by 90% within 45 minutes of ingesting the sugars. This makes it important to read labels to understand the amount of sugars, from a variety of possible sources, within a food product.

Protein

Definition: Protein makes up three-fourths of the dry weight of most cell matter and is involved in structures, hormones, enzymes, muscle contraction, immunologic response, and essential life functions. Macromolecules consisting of long sequences of amino acids [H2N–CHR–COOH] in peptide (amide).

Proteins are the basic building blocks from which bodily structures are formed. Protein is found in meats, fish, poultry, soy products, eggs, and dairy products. Protein should be consumed at every meal and snack and combined with fat and carbohydrate. To determine total daily protein requirement, take your weight and divide by 2.2 (this calculates your weight in kilograms). You should average approximately 1 gram of protein for each kilogram of weight. A 150-pound individual (150 divided by 2.2 equals 68 kilograms) would need approximately 68 grams of protein daily. Active individuals can eat up to 1½ grams of protein per kilogram of weight.

Red meat should be consumed at no more than 1/3 of your weekly meals. I encourage you to use lean cuts and avoid all ground beef and processed meat products. The concern about Mad Cow Disease has caused some to avoid all beef products. Because the infection is spread through brain/nervous and intestinal tissue, the chance of infection is negligible when you prepare whole labeled cuts of beef. If you want a hamburger, buy a whole piece of beef and have it ground by the butcher. Organic beef has been grown without antibiotics or hormone supplementation and has not been fed animal byproducts (the cause of Mad Cow Disease spread).

Purchase organic free-range chicken and non-farm raised fish when possible. Farm raised fish are fed enriched soy based feed including synthetic hormones. Fish pens circulate the water, but the fish are in an enclosed area with potentially higher concentrations of fecal matter. Wild fish are preferable but present their own set of problems. Higher concentrations of mercury have been found in canned tuna and fish that occupy the top of the food chain. These include: shark, halibut, and other large, dense meat fish. Generally, the smaller, younger fish are preferred for consumption.

Beef, chicken, and fish have 6 grams of protein for each ounce eaten. The average serving of this type protein is 3-5 ounces per meal.

Eggs are another excellent source of protein. Eggs received bad publicity as a result of the American Heart Association's concern for lowering cholesterol. Using a combination of whole eggs and egg whites can offset concern over cholesterol. One whole egg has 6 grams of protein. An egg white has 4 grams of protein. A 4-egg omelet (1 whole plus 3 whites) would count for 18 grams of protein.

Soy products can also be intermixed to meet the protein need. This includes: miso, natto, soymilk, tempeh, soy nuts, and defatted soy protein powder. There is concern with non-fermented soy products having a high concentration genistein. I recommend that you limit non-fermented soy to 1 serving every other day.

Dairy products, including cheeses, are another source of protein. Because full fat dairy products, higher in saturated fat, tend to be pro-inflammatory, I generally recommend a low-fat variety. Fermented dairy products (cottage cheese and yogurt) are tolerated well by individuals with lactose intolerance. ½ cup of cottage cheese has 12 grams of protein. The best cheeses, in addition to cottage cheese, are provolone, mozzarella, feta, fontina, goat, and ricotta.

Nuts and seeds are good sources for protein as well as fat. Almonds, pecans, black walnuts, peanuts, and cashews are some of the acceptable choices. Nuts and seeds should be eaten dry roasted or raw. Raw nuts should be soaked over night, the water poured off, and dried before eating.

Beans and rice, in combination, can count as a total protein. Each by itself does not contain the full complement of amino acids required for a total protein. When using rice and beans for a protein substitute, you need to take into account the glycemic load. A ½ cup serving should be combined with a 1 cup serving of a cruciferous vegetable to offset the insulin response.

For an excellent discussion on the affects of the various food groups on metabolism, I direct you to *The Schwarzbein Principle II—The Transition* by Diane Schwarzbein, MD. This text discusses the process of metabolic healing for individuals that may be insulin resistant and/or be experiencing adrenal exhaustion. Additionally, there are groupings of acceptable and unacceptable foods for the different categories.

Eating Right Without Freaking Out Over the Details!

I recommend the ratio of carbohydrates-proteins-fat to be 40%-30%-30% (of total daily calories), respectively. A reasonable recommendation for a female is to consume a total of 1200 to 1500 calories per day, depending on the level of activity. Ideally, each meal or snack you eat would have this ratio, but you do not have to do the math every time. Dr. Sears has developed what he refers to as the EYEBALL method. The tool necessary for the calculation is easily accessible—your hand!

Each meal begins with protein. The size of your hand is relative to the size of your body and, therefore, is an excellent guide to your protein needs. Your protein portion should equal the size and thickness of your palm. During your first few weeks of trying this eating plan, let your hand be your portion gauge.

Dr. Sears classifies carbohydrates as either favorable or unfavorable. Examples of the "most favorable" carbs are: asparagus, bean sprouts, broccoli, cabbage, various lettuces, greens, spinach, strawberries, blueberries, honeydew melon, cauliflower, and eggplant. Examples of "least favorite" are: bananas, beer, cake, candy bars, most juices, breads, carrots, cantaloupe, corn, honey, pasta, potatoes, rice, watermelon, and sugar. If you choose the favorable carbs, you get two large loose fists' worth. When you want carbs from the unfavorable list you get one tight fist's worth. The more favorable foods have a low "glycemic index" (see Appendix—B). That means, that as you digest them, they cause insulin to be secreted into the blood stream slowly and, therefore, keep your blood sugar levels stable. Higher glycemic index foods (starches, refined carbohydrates, and compact complex carbohydrates) will cause insulin to be secreted faster and in larger amounts resulting in fluctuation of your blood sugar.

The last nutrient is dietary fat. Balance out your meal by including a few nuts, olive oil, or olives. If your protein source is high in fat, you do not need to add more.

An easy way to start the balanced program is to divide your plate into thirds or fourths. In the first section of the plate put your palms' worth of protein. In the other two or three sections pick a fists' worth of vegetables and fruits to fill each section. Complete the meal by eating a salad with an oil and vinegar dressing. Additionally, use sliced nuts (lightly toasted almonds are excellent) to add protein to the salad.

Last is the reminder to eat five times per day—three meals and two snacks. Eat your first meal or snack within an hour of getting up. This is the area in which many individuals are deficient. Cereal, toast or bagel, orange juice, and coffee (the Standard American Diet—interestingly, combining the first letters spells the word SAD!) are an inefficient way to start the day. It is composed of mostly carbs and sugar, with little protein. Substitute ½ to ¾ cup cottage cheese with ½ to 1cup of fresh or frozen berries, a piece of whole grain toast with a nut butter or butter and olive oil combination. A combination of butter and canola oil (from Land-O-Lakes) can be purchased at many supermarkets. You can make your own by combining 2 sticks of butter with ¼ to ½ cup of extra virgin olive oil and refrigerating in an airtight container.

Actually mastering Zone eating requires a little more work (see *Entering the Zone* and other resources by Barry Sears, PhD.) The "zone" is built on food blocks. One "food block" contains a mini-block of carbohydrate, protein, and fat. The "block" value for various foods is detailed in the text. A meal for a female is generally 3 blocks, and for a male 4 blocks. Snacks are 1 block for each snack eaten (twice a day). A day's worth is 11 blocks for women and 14 blocks for men. Remember that the key to reaching the Zone is balancing carbohydrates, fats, and protein. Carbohydrates stimulate insulin secretion, and protein stimulates the production of glucagon (releasing stored sugar from the liver). The goal is to balance these two important hormones. Fat is thrown in to make your brain satisfied with your meal and to provide raw materials for the production of cellular hormones. For a complete explanation of Zone blocks and eating go to www.zoneperfect.com or read various texts by Dr. Barry Sears.

The End Result of Eating Run Amuck

There is no disputing the fact that Americans are fat and getting fatter. Total calorie consumption per individual is up. Three decades ago, 25% of the American population was considered overweight. Today, nearly 2/3 is overweight, with 30% of those labeled obese. The National Health and Nutrition Examination Survey (NHANES) indicated that in 1999-2000 64% of U.S. adults had a body mass index (BMI) at 25 or above. While this is a regrettable result of our lifestyle choices, the real disaster is the fact that ½ of American children are overweight. Statistics show that a 7-year old overweight female has an increased probability of early onset of puberty and an increased risk of breast cancer, Type II diabetes, and heart disease. Think of the reality; we have doomed our daughters to poor health, as adults, by the decisions made for them in childhood. While there are genetic issues that account for a minority of overweight children, remember that "genetics loads the gun, lifestyle pulls the trigger."

Our Attitude Toward Medicines

It has only been within the last century that synthetic medicines have been manufactured. Many current pharmaceuticals have a foundation in herbs and other natural materials. In our mind, we see the modern pharmacist counting out pills into an opaque plastic container. In reality, today's pharmacist is a significantly underutilized resource. Think about the last time you picked up a prescription, and the clerk asked you "do you have any questions for the pharmacist?" How many times have you actually discussed your medications with the individual (the pharmacist) who understands the actions and interactions of your medicines? We are aware that all prescribed medications have the potential for serious side effects, and yet, we generally take them without a clear understanding of their function. Of greater concern is our cavalier attitude toward over-the-counter (OTC) medications.

A common belief is that, just because the medications are not prescription, they are inherently safer. The indiscriminate use of non-steroidal anti-inflammatories (aspirin and NSAID's like ibuprofen, Advil, Aleve, etc.) is estimated to cause over 20,000 deaths per year, especially among the elderly. The average 70 year-old takes 7 prescription medications. If one of those is a blood thinner, utilizing aspirin and other ibuprofen type products increases the odds of gastric erosion and hemorrhage. Acetaminophen is associated with liver damage, and, in select individuals, even a small amount ingested with alcoholic beverages can lead to severe liver damage or death. The consumption of large amounts of Acetaminophen will cause irreversible liver damage and death. Whenever you start on a new medication, make a point of knowing why you are taking it, the possible side effects and contraindications, and for how long you need to take it. Every medicine, prescription or over-the-counter, comes with a tradeoff. Understand the benefits versus the risks. Discuss with the pharmacist ALL the medications you are taking, including herbal remedies. While herbs tend to have fewer side effects than synthetic prescription medications, they are medicines and can either increase or decrease the effects (of the prescription) if not used properly.

When the alternative exists, utilizing compounded medications tends to reduce the potential for over working the liver. Our liver is much like a large filter, responsible for cleaning unwanted or excess substances from our blood stream. Foods and medicines that pass through the stomach enter the blood by way of the hepatic (liver) portal system. As the substances pass through the intestinal lining, they are sent to the liver in what is referred to as "first pass." Liver activity metabolizes (breaks down) the substances. It then stores the metabolized substances, passes them into the systemic (body) circulation, or prepares them for elimination by way of the kidneys or bowels. In some cases, 90% of a medication is removed in this manner, and the remaining 10% is passed on. Synthetic medications have additional chemical properties (side chains). These side chains do not have an active function and must be removed from the structure of the drug. It is the liver's function to process the inactive side chains. Compounded medications, from a reputable pharmacist, are made in the same formula as that found "naturally" in the body. Because of this, the liver does not have to process the compounded drugs in the same manner. Even though they are referred to as "natural," it does not make them inherently any less dangerous; they are drugs and need to be utilized only as prescribed.

Food As Medicine

Earlier, I noted that nutrition includes everything that you put on and in your body. In like manner, you can consider everything that you put on and in your body as a medicine. The skin is the largest organ in the body. It is responsible for removing various substances from our body and is a method of introducing chemicals into the body. In past centuries, medications came from plants and flowers, herbs, and trees. The various concoctions were ingested or rubbed on the body. While we do not tend to think of our foods today as medicines, everything that we eat has to be processed by the body. The end result of that process, ultimately, will have an affect on cellular function. In most cases, the result may be so subtle that we are not aware of a perceptible change. On the other hand, you may have a rather marked reaction: increased pulse and urination (caffeine), energy (sugar), diarrhea and nausea (contaminated foods).

The carbohydrates, fats, and proteins that we eat are used to build our body's cells, utilized as energy, converted to hormones, or processed to meet the other needs of body function. As noted previously, foods that are organic and minimally processed provide the body with the needed building substances in as pure a form as possible. Much like the processing of medications, the liver must deal with carbohydrates, fats, and proteins in a similar manner. When the foodstuffs are contaminated with residual chemicals (pesticides, fertilizers, hormones, etc.), the liver completes a process termed biotransformation—packaging the substance for removal from the body. One healthy goal is not to overtax the liver's function. Many times you may hear the argument that organic produce and meats are no better than non-organic. The contention is that you do not get more from the organic over the non-organic foodstuffs. That statement is essentially true. What is important to understand, is that it is not what you get from organic, it is what you DO NOT get! In the last century it is estimated that over 30,000 chemicals have been manufactured and introduced into the food chain and environment. While there is minimal conclusive evidence that the majority of these chemicals are harmful by themselves to the body, concern is mounting about repeated long-term exposure and the effect of the combining of substances.

Our current healthcare system needs to place more value on understanding the effects of bodily exposure to these thousands of chemicals. At the center of the problem is the model of healthcare practiced today in America.

Functional medicine is a comprehensive system of health management based on a *"Health Model."* H. L. "Sam" Queen, CCN, of the Institute for Health Realities states that health is best attained by supporting the body's design for keeping itself well. Every attempt is made to address issues of health and disease in a specific order of importance. The *"Disease Model"* (rescue medicine) is founded on the belief that lowering the incidence of disease, infection, and health risk factors attains health.

Physicians and scientists are often referred to as reductionists. This means that the goal of their studies is to reduce the problem being investigated to the lowest common denominator. One initial concept was that the brain controlled all bodily function. Due to the inter-connectiveness of hormonal and cellular function it is now known that the brain works in concert with, not dictatorially over, other physiological systems. Final control is not linear, that is, going from A to B to C in a definite order. Rather, the body collects and directs information randomly, much like the Internet processing data through multiple routers. Therefore, it is possible to approach health issues by determining the systems, which when altered, would have the greatest affect on the body as a whole (see "A New Paradigm").

Sam Queen has developed a system called the *BioDesign Model of Health*. It is based on addressing specific subclinical defects and other clinical factors. Correction, of these areas first, will result in the reduction of disease, infection, and risk factors.

Sam W. came to the office concerned over pain and tingling in both hands and feet. He noted that a few days earlier he had awoken out of a dead sleep with what he described as sharp, ice pick, sticking pain that felt like his arms and legs had been immersed in ice water. Subsequent MRI of the head and brain, neck and low back where inconclusive, other than marked disc degeneration. Electrical studies (EMG) of the arms and legs noted carpal and tarsal tunnel syndrome but nothing helpful in determining the cause of his symptoms. Medical recommendations included anti-inflammatories and narcotic medication for pain control. Using the *BioDesign* format of evaluation he was tested for inflammatory tendencies, glucose and insulin levels, and acid-base balance. When initial treatment protocols did not result in consistent improvement, he underwent genetic testing for inflammatory markers. These tests revealed a genetic alteration in the production of prostaglandins. It is known that the omega-3 essential fatty acids (EFA's) are anti-inflammatory. It was discovered that one segment of his omega-3's was preferentially affecting the synthesis of the prostaglandin PGE2 from arachidonic acid in the omega-6 chain. Previously, Sam had been treated with 8-10 grams of omega-3's per day. Instead of increasing the anti-inflammatory effect, it was increasing the production of inflammatory chemicals. Sam was placed on a balance of omega-3 (2-4 grams) and omega-6 supplementation, a balanced diet with limited simple carbohydrates, and the admonition to eat protein and good fats with every meal or snack. This date he notes marked improvement. He has some episodes of pain ranging from a freezing sensation to pinpricks if he eats a meal high in carbohydrates or when under periods of stress. Both of these influences result in elevated insulin production. The elevated insulin was another factor revealed with testing that affected the essential fatty acid synthesis. In the end, through using the *BioDesign Model* of evaluation, we were able to pinpoint the cause of the pain and treat it.

Think of the *Disease Model* of health as an army that identifies (and names) battles, often on a number of fronts at the same time. The goal is to win the battle and then rest, waiting to possibly fight that same battle again. Minimal or no effort is given to understanding the reason for the war in the first place. Our current approach to heart disease is a good example. Minimal efforts are made to change a lifestyle that leads to cardiovascular disease. The most visible attempt to prevent heart disease is in monitoring cholesterol. The typical approach is to recommend, initially, a low-fat diet and exercise, followed by the use of lipid lowering medications. Many physicians make an effort to address weight and smoking but really have received little to no actual training in effectively modifying these concerns. Failure of these measures may result in a patient undergoing a cardiac catheterization with stint placement or bypass surgery to open occluded heart arteries.

Currently, there are few programs of post-surgical intervention that are effective. Too often a patient will have a second heart surgery within a 1-5 year period. Health insurers generally fail to pay for programs that develop individualized intervention programs. Frequently, the programs "handed out" are based on generalized recommendations that do not take into consideration the physiological differences of the patient.

State-of-the-art diagnostic procedures and high cost surgical procedures are thought to be the answer to our diseased conditions. The area for battle is identified, labeled, and a battle plan developed and executed. More efforts need to be made to identify the underlying reason for the system failure. While many doctors are beginning to approach health in this manner, the success will lie in patient compliance. It is the individual's (patient's) ultimate responsibility to change negative lifestyle choices. The reason that health insurers do not pay for the needed programs is that they do not see a positive association between these plans of intervention and reduced healthcare cost. In summary, these plans too often fail because they are not individualized, based on ineffective physiological intervention, and a lack of patient compliance.

Remember the statement, *"medicine is what the doctor does for you, health is what you do for yourself."* Until you understand the importance of that statement, you will continue to fail in repeated attempts to "get well." You need to listen to the subtle changes in your body and to understand the signs and symptoms that require immediate attention.

Physicians that practice functional medicine are trained to note these subtle changes and develop lifestyle interventions. This approach includes an awareness of numerous medical issues:

1. Subclinical defects including:
   a. pH balance—acid/base
   b. Free calcium
   c. Anaerobic metabolism
   d. Chronic inflammation
   e. Oxidative stress
   f. Connective tissue breakdown
2. Evaluation of toxic exposure (see Section 2)
3. Prognostic indicators
4. Risk factors' identification
5. Infection
6. Disease management

Note: above, that the foundational elements of the Disease Model of Health are numbers 4, 5, and 6. The proper approach to attaining and maintaining health is in correcting the first 3 areas.

How This Applies to You!

pH balance: most Americans eat a diet that tends to result in the blood, saliva, urine, and cellular fluids being too acidic. While you cannot easily monitor the blood and cells, it is inexpensive and easy to monitor the pH of your saliva and urine. You can purchase Hydrion paper (remember the blue and red litmus paper in high school science class) from a pharmacy. Ideally, both the urine and saliva should be 7.0. It is acceptable for urine to range from 6.0 to 7.5, and saliva from 6.5 to 7.5 (this may vary depending on the time of day). A pH of 5.5 or below in the urine, and 6.0 or below in saliva, indicates an acidic state that needs to be addressed. You can raise your pH by:

1. Breathing deep—raise your arms while inhaling, lower them as you exhale.
2. Add weak acids to your diet—citric acid from lemons and limes, lactic acid from cultured dairy products (plain yogurt and cottage cheese), malic acid from apples and apple cider, and acetic acid in vinegar.
3. Mild to moderate exercise.
4. Supplementation with glutamine and phosphorus. This should only be undertaken under the supervision of a physician who understands the proper dosage and form of supplementation.

You can make a few generalized assumptions from basic lab results. (You should always get a copy of all blood tests for your records).

- A healthy ratio of sodium (average around 140 mg/dl) to chloride (average 100 mg/dl) is 1.4 to 1. A ratio of 1.33 to 1, or below, indicates an acid condition. Eat more frequently, especially if you are under stress. While 1 tsp of baking soda can correct this, I do not recommend that you attempt this unsupervised.

- A carbon dioxide reading below 23 mg/dl may indicate a lack of weak acid production by the pancreas or a deficiency of protein enzymes in the stomach. Follow the initial recommendations for correcting pH.

- An albumin reading below 4.0 generally indicates chronic inflammation.

Albumin is a protein that acts as the body's main acid sponge. It is an important part of immune response and hormone transport. Coupled with a total protein below 7.0 or above 7.6 indicates protein deficiency or poor protein utilization.

- A Total Protein (TP) below 7.0 generally indicates that you are not digesting protein through the gastrointestinal system efficiently. This can be improved by using a proteolytic enzyme (improving digestion of protein) at mealtime. If you have a history of gastric ulcer, do not use an enzyme that has hydrochloric acid in it, unless supervised by a physician. Take the supplement between 15 minutes before and up to the start of the meal.

- A Total Protein over 7.6 indicates that you are not efficiently recycling the protein that you have digested. This can be addressed by taking the proteolytic enzyme between meals on an empty stomach. Common proteolytic enzymes are pepsin and papain. The use of trypsin and chymotrypsin should be supervised, especially if you have a history of panceatitis.

The subclinical actions of digestion and colon/bowel health are an overlooked area. In evaluating bowel movements, they should be well formed, not overly odiferous, and occur 1 to 2 times per day. One of the frequently seen conditions in medical practices today is GERD (gastrointestinal esophageal reflux disease). The usual treatment is to take one of the medications directed toward reducing acid production. Too often, the problem is not an over production of acid, but inefficient digestion. This is commonly associated with a lack of hydrochloric acid (HCl) at the time of ingestion of food. Utilizing a full spectrum digestive enzyme with supplemental HCl, generally, makes a significant difference in the feeling of bloating, gas, and burning. The digestive enzyme should include pepsin, papain, pancreatin, and amylase, in addition to betaine HCl (hydrochloric acid). As previously noted, this should be taken approximately 15 minutes before the meal. To offset burning and pain between meals, eat high protein snacks mid-morning and mid-afternoon. A mixture of Knox gelatin made with unfiltered apple juice or Concorde grape juice is an excellent protein source.

To improve bowel function, you need to promote the growth of "good" bacteria. An overgrowth of "bad" bacteria leads to increased anaerobic activity, increased acidity, and toxicity. Improvement can be accomplished by using the "mucosa builder" (the mucosa is the lining of the intestine that transports the digested foods from inside the intestine to the blood stream). The formula for the "mucosa builder" can be found in Appendix C. It is a combination of extra virgin olive oil, salted butter, probiotics (the "good" bacteria), and raw honey (for the bacteria to feed on). Let the butter slightly soften and then place in the blender with the olive oil and blend. Add the probiotics by opening the capsules and pouring it into the mixture. Add the honey and blend smooth. Place the mixture in a glass container that closes tight. For the next 2 weeks, use 1 tablespoon of the mixture at breakfast. If you find taking it off a spoon objectionable, it is OK to spread it on toast. I have found that an olive oil that has been infused with lemon or lime makes the spread tasty (an excellent brand of infused olive oils can be found at Williams-Sonoma). After the initial 2-week period, continue to use ½ to 1 tablespoon of this spread 3 times per week. Additionally, it is good to make a butter spread of ¼ cup olive oil to 2 sticks of butter to use on a regular basis in place of plain butter. Olive oil is an omega-9 fat and, except for calories, has only positive effects on the body, unless ingested in very high quantities.

Your Inflammatory Status

Knowing your body's inflammatory status is as important, if not more so, than knowing your cholesterol numbers. Half of all heart attacks occur in individuals with normal cholesterol levels. With the constant barrage of advertising related to cholesterol lowering medications, individuals have a fairly good idea whether their total cholesterol, HDL and LDL, are within an acceptable range. As previously noted, lowering your cholesterol with medication, unfortunately, does not guarantee improved health. In fact, your cholesterol will rise in response to chronic inflammation in an effort to protect the brain and other neurological tissues. Artificially lowering this response may lead to additional health problems, especially if the rise was a result of exposure to toxic substances (mercury, petroleum exposure, pesticides, etc). When attempting to lower cholesterol, it must be done in association with a thorough inflammatory evaluation. Failing other measures, when utilizing a statin type medication becomes necessary, it has been revealed that part of its effectiveness is in its anti-inflammatory properties.

The relationship to cardiovascular health and inflammation is especially relevant for women. Remember that heart attacks for a woman are a combination of minor arterial plaguing and spasm. Both of these factors are related to an increased state of inflammation.

In a nutshell, by design, inflammation is a lifesaver. It is part of the body's ability to respond to injury, infection (bacterial, viral, parasitic), and other damaging physical insults. This is a highly refined, orchestrated response—one that ideally knows when to start and when to shut down. As a result of varying circumstances, the body's ability to control the inflammatory response may not shut down when appropriate. The end result is a state of chronic inflammation. Chronic inflammation, in association with elevated levels of free iron and calcium, ultimately leads to increased connective tissue degeneration—arthritis, autoimmune diseases including lupus, fibromyalgia, multiple sclerosis—and accelerated cardiovascular disease, stroke, and Alzheimer's disease.

Dr. Peter Libby, Chief of Cardiovascular Medicine at Brigham and Women's Hospital in Boston, notes that "the strategies our bodies used for survival were important in a time when we didn't have processing plants to purify our water, when we didn't have sewers to protect us." These evolutionary strategies included "our ability to fight off microbial invaders." It has been speculated that a number of our lifestyle choices, in addition to our living longer, have led to chronic bodily inflammation, the body's inability to moderate or shut off a normal function. These lifestyle changes include: diets high in sugar, refined carbohydrates, and saturated fats, little or no exercise, and elevated levels of cortisol from chronic stress.

From a holistic healthcare point of view, one of the common signs of inflammation, fever, needs to be appreciated. Fever is generally the result of an acute injury or bodily insult. Too often the first thing done at the onset of fever is to reach for one of the over-the-counter remedies. In this case, it is assumed that by decreasing the fever (which is done as a measure of comfort), that the "cause" has been removed. In reality, inappropriately lowering the body's initial response will prolong and delay the natural reparative process. Fever is associated with activation of a number of immune responses (macrophages, mast cells, cytokines)—it causes one to rest and reduce the body's energy output. Prolonged elevations of fever (greater than 102 F in adults and 104 F in children) need to be addressed medically as an indicator of possible bacterial infection.

A simple method for evaluating an individual's inflammatory status is with a blood test—C-Reactive Protein—CRP. While the CRP is a generalized test, there is a heart sensitive component referred to as hsCRP (high sensitivity). In February 2003, the American Heart Association and the Center for Disease Control (CDC) jointly endorsed guidelines for its use. In recent studies of 28,000 patients, it was found that individuals with the highest CRP were four (4) times more likely to have a heart attack (MI - myocardial infarction) and three (3) times more likely to have a stroke. Early evaluation of CRP has been found to be a reliable predictor in signifying risk of heart disease, stroke, and adult onset diabetes.

Researchers are now aware that heart disease is not simply a "plumbing" problem. This is especially true for the female population where atherosclerotic buildup is not the major factor or predictor of heart attack. Research on the relationship of inflammation has markedly increased over the last few years. Dr. Paul Ridker, a cardiologist at Brigham and Women's Hospital, notes "the whole field of inflammation research is about to explode." This has been the result of secondary findings related to other drug treatments. In 2000, researchers noted that patients taking Celebrex for treatment of arthritis had a reduced tendency to develop intestinal polyps (precancerous growths). This has prompted additional research into the relationship of inflammation to breast cancer, Alzheimer's and other memory loss conditions, and ALS (Lou Gehrig's disease). Current medical protocol for elevated CRP includes the daily use of low dose (81 g) aspirin, a commonly used anti-inflammatory. This is providing researchers with a large database to evaluate the use of aspirin in relation to development of the previously noted diseases. It should be noted that the indiscriminate use of all anti-inflammatory medications, including over-the-counter (aspirin, ibuprofen, Advil, Aleve, Nuprin), results in approximately 20,000 deaths a year. These deaths are related to gastrointestinal bleeding/hemorrhage. Care should always be taken when utilizing anti-inflammatory medications in association with blood thinners or with a history of stomach or intestinal ulceration. While anti-inflammatory medications initially control inflammatory response, of greater importance is uncovering and treating the cause of the inflammation. In general, the standard American diet is pro-inflammatory, resulting in a urinary and saliva pH less than 6.0 (please refer to the previous section—Food As Medicine—for evaluating and treating chronic inflammation).

While chronic inflammation is associated with all degenerative diseases, it is an understanding of the relationship to cardiovascular disease that may unlock significant changes in treatment protocols. Previous treatment has been focused on the fatty buildup found in the lining of arteries, especially arteries of the heart. A certain portion of LDL cholesterol (bad cholesterol) has been identified as the major supplier of raw materials for these deposits. This portion is referred to as oxidized LDL cholesterol and results from increased cellular oxidation and free radical production. Ingestion of certain types of food, including products made from powdered milk and creamers, trans fats, rancid oils, sugar and alcohol, will increase this action. Exposure to cigarette smoke, petroleum distillates, and other environmental endocrine disruptors (ED) also increases free radical production. Arterial deposits become unstable in the presence of elevated homocysteine and chronic inflammation.

General measures to control chronic inflammation:

·   Utilize a pharmaceutical grade fish oil daily—1 to 4 grams per day.
·   Decrease the intake of sugar, alcohol, and refined carbohydrates.
·   Increase consumption of cruciferous vegetables (see glossary for a list).
·   Restrict full fat dairy products while eating a daily serving of low-fat cultured dairy (plain yogurt or cottage cheese).
·   Eat an apple per day—including the skin.
·   Eliminate sources of partially hydrogenated and trans fats.
·   Use fresh lemon or lime in water to promote improved acid-base balance.
·   If you are on a low carb diet, supplement with folic acid in a multiple vitamin to control possible elevated levels of homocysteine.

Part Seven

Putting It All Together

Now, with God's help, I shall become myself.
—Soren Kierkegaard

An Overview

We have covered a lot of ground in the previous chapters. Remember in the beginning, I promised to K.I.S.S. (keep it simple stupid). At this point, the information may have started to run together, and you are left with that "what's the use" feeling. As you are aware, there are a lot of books available that cover the issues of women's health, hormones, weight loss, and other current medical issues relevant to the female population. Now comes the time when we will see if I can help you make a difference, one that will last a lifetime.

The items listed under "Foundational Concepts," and Parts 1 and 2 are *imperatives*. Introduce these points into your life *now*. Make arrangements with your physician (or find a new physician) to get necessary tests completed. The points in Parts 3 through 6 can be applied as you see fit, but I have listed them in what I believe is the best order. Review the recommendations in Chapters 3 (Let's Get Started) and 14 (Step by Step). The difference here is in PROGRESSIVE PRACTICAL APPLICATION.

Foundational Concepts

Let's review a few basic foundational concepts:

1. Medicine is what the doctor can do for you; health is what you can do for yourself.
2. You have an important role in your healthcare choices.
3. Our goal is health and wellness.
4. Health is not the absence of symptoms and disease.
5. The road to improved health will take time and involve lifestyle changes—there are NO short cuts!

Part 1—Application

1. Get a baseline physical with a physician with whom you trust and can develop a "doctor-patient partnership."
2. When age appropriate, get mammograms, PAP smears, and screening for colorectal cancer and bone density (DEXA scan).
3. Learn how to perform a self-breast exam—become comfortable with your anatomy (see Appendix—I).
4. Know your personal family medical history and how it relates to the risk factors for breast cancer and heart disease.
5. Quit smoking.

Part 2—Application

1. Understand that regaining health is *About Being Complete*: (A) About—it's OK to make your health a priority; (B) Being—living in today, without guilt of the past or fear of the future; (C) Complete—a balance of mind, body, and spirit.
2. Write down the *plan* for your health. Have an accountability partner to help you work this plan.
3. Start with one positive step and build on your successes. Do not be afraid of failure. When things do not work out the way you intended, consider it a detour, another opportunity to succeed.
4. Knowing your genetic predispositions can help you effectively map out

a plan for improved health.

5. Try to make the most out of your lifestyle change efforts. Make positive, progressive choices that will give you the most bang-for-your-buck (and time!)

6. Do not believe everything you see advertised.

Part 3—Application

1. Understand the goal of stress reduction is to balance your hormonal systems by becoming more comfortable "within your own skin."

2. Practice a stress reduction exercise.

3. Sleep better. Recent studies reveal that the majority of Americans are sleep deprived. This step is intimately related to prioritizing your activities. Remember the ABC's! The short-term use of 1-2 mg. of melatonin taken prior to bedtime can help. If this continues to be a problem, having your a.m. cortisol level checked is appropriate.

4. Exercise on a regular basis. If you can do nothing else: walk at lunch; park farther from the office or store; take the stairs when possible.

5. Organize your personal environment—both at home and at work.

6. Plan "downtime." Start reading a book for pleasure (not work related) before bed.

7. Plan a "date day." Having something to look forward to during a hectic week can be energizing.

8. If you are a "reactive, shoot from the hip" kind of person, make a list of what irritates you. Anticipate your response to situations; know how you will act when that particular "irritant" presents itself again.

Part 4—Application

1. Understand that the goal of this section is to decrease the amount of exposure to various types of chemicals that: 1) mimic the effects of estrogen, and 2) interrupt the normal function of cellular receptors (endocrine disruptors—EDs).

2. Do not smoke and minimize exposure to second-hand smoke.

3. Start to shop and eat organic. The simplest, first step, (if you or your family drinks milk), is to purchase organic dairy products. Most major supermarkets have a selection of these items.

4. Check your kitchen, makeup, and bath products. Buy from a company that uses environmentally sensitive and safe goods.

5. Avoid all personal body care products that contain petrochemicals (petroleum based).

6. Download a copy of "The Cosmetic Ingredients Reference Guide & Dictionary."
7. If you work around petroleum based products, pesticides, fertilizers, and other potentially toxin chemicals, take measures to protect yourself. Use respirators and protective coverings when handling these materials.
8. Eat lower on the food chain, including wild, deep-water fish.
9. Eat fewer processed foods and do not heat foods in plastic containers.

Part 5—Application

1. Understand the goal is to decrease your exposure to exogenous (outside sources) of estrogen.
2. If you are on chemical birth control (pills or patch) that contains estrogens and progestins, you can never balance your hormones until you discontinue their use. Natural Family Planning (NFP - see Appendix H) can be highly effective when utilized as taught. This takes time and extra effort, but the benefit to your body makes it worth considering.
3. If you are considering estrogen (ERT) or hormone replacement therapy (HRT) get your estrogen, progesterone, and testosterone levels checked in advance. The only reason to supplement these is to keep the body's level of hormones at a normal, physiological level. That is: not too much; not too little. If you decide that hormone replacement is appropriate, use natural, bioidentical hormones from a compounding pharmacy.
4. Topical progesterone may be appropriate for pre-menopausal and menopausal symptoms (see "Part—5 Practical Application" for usage instructions).
5. Read the studies (see "What the Studies Say"). Every medical treatment comes with benefits and risk. It is your responsibility to try to understand the benefit versus the risk so that you can make an informed choice. I have succeeded in improving your overall health if you now understand the importance of gaining and then applying knowledge.

Part 6—Application

1. The goal for proper nutrition is to give your body the proper type and amount of foods to produce fuel, building blocks, and neurotransmitters. In essence, think of everything that goes into your mouth as affecting one or more of these areas.
2. The balance of carbohydrates, proteins, and fats, along with portion control, is the heart of every successful eating program. Your eating habits control insulin production/balance, and the body's inflammatory

responses. Know which foods affect the rise of insulin (see Appendix—B) and inflammation (see "Your Inflammatory Status" and *Cruciferous* in the glossary).

3. Eat a balanced breakfast. American breakfasts (when eaten) tend to be primarily carbohydrates. Eat within 1 hour of getting up.

4. Eat mid-morning and mid-afternoon snacks that include protein and good fat. Eat before you get hungry. If you are aware of hunger, it generally indicates that your blood sugar has dropped.

5. Pick foods that are higher in fiber.

6. Start a basic supplementation program (see Appendix—D).

7. Become a label reader. Know what is in your food.

8. Avoid "fast-food" type restaurants. If you must eat at one of the major chains, check www.zoneperfect.com for a list of acceptable fare. Remember that the "low carb" choices are not necessarily low calorie (think bad fat).

Final Thoughts

Someone wrote that luck is when preparation meets opportunity. So, as luck would have it, in the preparation of this manuscript I had the opportunity to confer with a number of gifted individuals, who challenged me in my writing. As a result, I believe that *What's a Woman to Do?* is but a beginning in the quest to help women achieve improved health. *What's a Woman to Do?* primarily addresses health issues for women in their early thirties to late fifties. During the research of the four focus areas, it was evident that there was additional important information that needed to be brought to women's attention. It starts with the decisions made for us in our early years and continues to those that we as adults make. During our lives each of us experiences three types of relationships. First, are those individuals who mentor us; second, those who we walk beside in our daily lives; and finally, those that, by actions and decisions, we mentor. We must take health related decisions seriously, as they have profound effects not just on oneself, but on those we are in relationship with.

In a follow-up text due out in 2005, *7 to 70: Decades of Womanhood,* Dr. Linda Miles, psychotherapist, and myself will parallel the psychological and physical development of a woman from childhood through the latter years. Following the "About Being Complete" and "Progressive Practical Application" format, we give real-life methods in dealing with physical and mental health issues that affect every female. Current research validates the fact that "all illness, if not psychosomatic in foundation, has a definite psychosomatic component." In *The Molecules of Emotion*, the author continues by stating, "the molecules of our emotions share intimate connections with, and indeed are inseparable from, our physiology." Dr. Miles and I will bring these scientific truths to a reality for practical application in your life.

Appendix A—Body Mass Index

Definition: an anthropometric measure of body mass, defined as weight in kilograms divided by height in meters squared; a method of determining caloric nutritional status.

The BMI (Body Mass Index) is an index of "fatness." In the original Framingham Heart Study, there was a positive relationship between BMI and cardiovascular health and glucose intolerance. For women, the desirable BMI is 21-23 kg/m2.

How to interpret your BMI:

18 or less = underweight
19-24 = weight appropriate
25-29 = overweight
30 and above = obese

Your goal: to keep your weight in the 19 to 24 range.

The Centers for Disease Control maintains a website with relevant information at: www.cdc.gov/nccdphp/dnpa/bmi/calc-bmi.htm. There is an area of discussion on body shape and metabolic syndrome.

For additional information on BMI see www.halls.md. Included is information on breast cancer (risk assessment) and ideal weight calculations (relative to your age, height, and current weight).

Body Mass Index
Height—feet & inches

Weight	5'0"	5'1"	5'2"	5'3"	5'4"	5'5"	5'6"	5'7"
100	20	19	18	18	17	17	16	16
105	21	20	19	19	18	17	17	16
110	21	21	20	19	19	18	18	17
115	22	22	21	20	20	19	19	18
120	23	23	22	21	21	20	19	19
125	24	24	23	22	21	21	20	20
130	25	25	24	23	22	22	21	20
135	26	26	25	24	23	22	22	21
140	27	26	26	25	24	23	23	22
145	28	27	27	26	25	24	23	23
150	29	28	27	27	26	25	24	23
155	30	29	28	27	27	26	25	24
160	31	30	29	28	27	27	26	25
165	32	31	30	29	28	27	27	26
170	33	32	31	30	29	28	27	27
175	34	33	32	31	30	29	28	27
180	35	34	33	32	31	30	29	28
185	36	35	34	33	32	31	30	29
190	37	36	35	34	33	32	31	30
195	38	37	36	35	33	32	31	31
200	39	38	37	35	34	33	32	31
205	40	39	37	36	35	34	33	32
210	41	40	38	37	36	35	34	33
215	42	41	39	38	37	36	35	34
220	43	42	40	39	38	37	36	34
225	44	43	41	40	39	37	36	35
230	45	43	42	41	39	38	37	36
235	46	44	43	42	40	39	38	37
240	47	45	44	43	41	40	39	38
245	48	46	45	43	42	41	40	38
250	49	47	46	44	43	42	40	39

Body Mass Index
Height—feet & inches

Weight	5'8"	5'9"	5'10	5'11	6'0"	6'1"	6'2"	6'3"
100	15	15	14	14	14	13	13	12
105	16	16	15	15	14	14	13	13
110	17	16	16	15	15	15	14	14
115	17	17	17	16	16	15	15	14
120	18	18	17	17	16	16	15	15
125	19	18	18	17	17	16	16	16
130	20	19	19	18	18	17	17	17
135	21	20	19	19	18	18	17	17
140	21	21	20	20	19	18	18	17
145	22	21	21	20	20	19	19	18
150	23	22	22	21	20	20	20	19
155	24	23	22	22	21	20	20	19
160	24	24	23	22	22	21	21	20
165	25	24	24	23	22	22	21	21
170	26	25	24	24	23	22	22	21
175	27	26	25	24	24	23	22	22
180	27	27	26	25	24	24	23	22
185	28	27	27	26	25	24	24	23
190	29	28	27	26	26	25	24	24
195	30	29	28	27	26	26	25	24
200	30	30	29	28	27	26	26	25
205	31	30	29	29	28	27	26	26
210	32	31	30	29	28	28	27	26
215	33	32	31	30	29	28	28	27
220	33	32	32	31	30	29	28	27
225	34	33	32	31	31	30	29	28
230	35	34	33	32	31	30	30	29
235	36	35	34	33	32	31	30	29
240	36	35	34	33	33	32	31	30
245	37	36	35	34	33	32	31	31
250	38	37	36	35	34	33	32	31

Appendix B—Glycemic Food List

In understanding glycemic index and glycemic load, it is first important to understand exactly what they are and how they affect our metabolism.

Glycemic Index: The Glycemic Index (GI) is the relative rate that carbohydrates enter the blood stream and the corresponding rise in insulin. Three factors need to be included in determining the glycemic index: 1) the amount of fiber contained, 2) the amount of fat (the higher the fat content, the slower the digestion rate), and 3) the composition of the carbohydrate (a higher glucose content equals a higher GI, while a higher fructose content equals a lower GI. Fructose has to be converted to glucose in the liver, a relatively slow process). The concept of glycemic index was a major improvement in the dietary field but did not work well with low-density carbohydrates. This was resolved with the calculation of glycemic load.

Glycemic Load: the Glycemic Load (GL) is the glycemic index value divided by 100 and multiplied by its available carbohydrate content (in grams). Carbohydrate content is total carbohydrate (grams) minus the available fiber (grams). The illustration below shows that it takes over 12 cups of broccoli to equal the insulin stimulating effect of 1 cup of pasta.

Food	Volume	Total (grams)	Carb (grams)	Fiber Insulin stimulating carbs - grams
Pasta	1 cup (cooked)	40	2	38
Apple	1 medium	20	4	16
Broccoli	1 cup	7	4	3

Information from: *The Omega Rx Zone*, Barry Sears, PhD.

There are numerous ways to classify foods with regard to their level of glycemic index. Barry Sears, Ph.D., classifies them as "favorable," "less favorable," and "unacceptable" (for a complete list, including recipes and an e-mail update service, go to www.zoneperfect.com). In the *South Beach Diet,* these foods are listed as low GI (14 to 54), medium (55 to 70), and high (71 to 103).

A brief list of foods, by type, and their glycemic indexes follows:

RICE AND GRAINS

Barley	25
Converted, White Rice	38
Buckwheat	54
Brown Rice	55
Basmati Rice	58
Couscous	65
Cornmeal	68
Short Grain, White Rice	72
Wild Rice	87
Instant, White Rice	87

DAIRY

Yogurt, Artificially Sweetened	14
Whole Milk	31
Skim Milk	32
Yogurt, Sweetened	33
Ice Cream, Premium	38
Ice Cream, Low Fat	43

JUICES

Tomato	38
Apple	40
Pineapple	46
Grapefruit	48
Orange	53

BREADS

Pumpernickel	41
Sourdough	53
Stone Ground Whole Wheat	53
Pita, Whole Wheat	57
Whole Meal Rye	58
White	69
Bagel	72

PASTA

Fettuccini	32
Spaghetti, Whole Wheat	37
Spaghetti, White	38
Capellini	45
Linguine	46
Macaroni	47

CRACKERS

Stoned Wheat Thins	67
Melba Toast	70
Kavli Crispbread	71
(Saltine Type) Crackers	74
Graham Crackers	74
Water Crackers	78
Rice Cakes	82

VEGETABLES & FRUITS

Broccoli	10
Cabbage	10
Lettuce	10
Mushrooms	10
Onions	10
Red Peppers	10
Asparagus	15
Zucchini	15
Green Beans	15
Lettuce (all varieties)	15
Tomatoes	15
Spinach	15
Grapefruit	25
Apricots (dried)	31
Apples	38
Pears	38
Plums	39
Peaches	42
Oranges	44
Pineapple Juice	46
Grapes	46
Green Peas	48
Carrots	49

Corn, fresh	60
Beets	64
Pumpkin	75
Parsnips	97

SWEETENERS

Fructose	20
Table Sugar	65
Honey	75

MISCELLANEOUS

Popcorn	55
Pizza, Cheese	60
Mars Bar	64
Angel Cake	67
Mashed Potatoes	70

Appendix C—Mucosa Builder

½ cup extra virgin olive oil (can use lemon or orange infused)
1 stick salted or lightly salted butter
10 capsules of acidophilus /lactobacillus (probiotic)
1 tablespoon raw honey

Allow the butter to soften slightly and blend with the olive oil. Add the honey and probiotics and blend smooth. Put mixture in an airtight container and refrigerate.

Use 1 tablespoon per day for 2 weeks. If you find the taste or texture difficult to swallow, spread the mixture on a piece of whole grain toast at your AM meal.

After 2 weeks, continue to use 2-3 times per week.

This is going to help rebuild your intestinal lining and assist in efficient absorption of food and improved bowel movements.

The Mucosa Builder formula is a product of the Institute for Health Realities, Colorado Springs, Colorado.

Appendix D—Supplementation

The American Medical Association currently recommends that all adults take a multiple vitamin. Due to the processing of foods, increased free radicals resulting from environmental exposure, and stress, I recommend that the average female take the following supplements:

- MULTIVITAMIN: 1-2 tablets daily per label recommendation.
- OMEGA-3 FATTY ACIDS: 1 gram (1000 milligrams), 2—3 times a day (anti-inflammatory).
- VITAMIN E: 400-800 IU daily (antioxidant)
- VITAMIN C: 1 gram (1000 milligrams) 1-2 times per day (free radical scavenger).
- VITAMIN B COMPLEX: 50 mg daily (for stress).
- CALCIUM: 1000-1500 mg daily - with magnesium (2:1 ratio) & vitamin D. I recommend calcium citrate when supplemental calcium is needed, as it is the most digestible at commonly found pH levels.
- BROMELAIN: 500 –1000 mg, 2 times daily between meals (to fight inflammation).
- COENZYME Q10: 60 to 100 mg daily (100 mg if taking a lipid lowering statin drug).
- ALPHA LIPOIC ACID: 50-100 mg daily (antioxidant).

Actual dosages may vary and additional supplements prescribed based on clinical findings.

Appendix E—Thyroid Test

A commonly used laboratory test for evaluating thyroid function is measurement of TSH (thyroid stimulating hormone). A normal value for this test varies slightly from lab to lab but, generally, is in the range of .35 to 5.5 mIU/L. You can evaluate thyroid function with a home test, measurement of basal body temperature (BBT), which will give a general indication for hypothyroidism (decreased thyroid function).

Prior to the onset of menstruation and after menopause, the test can be conducted on any day of the month. For menstruating females, the test is most effective when conducted 2 to 3 days after the onset of the period.

Directions:

Shake down an oral thermometer before retiring for bed and place conveniently next to the bed.

On awakening, before getting out of bed, place the thermometer snuggly in the armpit for 10 minutes. It is important that the thermometer remain in place for a full 10 minutes. It is also important that the test be completed prior to activity.

Record the temperature and compare it to the temperatures below. I recommend that you complete the test on at least three consecutive days. The test may be an early indication of infection; therefore, the test is invalid (with regard to thyroid function) if you become ill in the next few days.

The following temperatures are a general guideline:

· Normal temperature: 97.8 to 98.2 F.
· Less than 97.2 F may indicate decreased thyroid function.
· Greater than 98.2 F may indicate possible infection.

From: *Hypothyroidism, the Unsuspected Illness*, Bioda Barnes, MD, Lawrence Galton, Harper & Row Publishing, 1976.

Additional laboratory tests, in addition to TSH, that may add insight with regard to thyroid function, include: T3, reverse T3 (rT3), T7, and thyroid antibody test.

Appendix F—Trans Fat-Free Zone

Trans fat or partially hydrogenated fats are the result of a manufacturing process where hydrogen is forced through liquid oils. It shows up in the cooking of french fries and other fried foods, and in the manufacturing of cookies, crackers, potato chips, margarines, and salad dressings. In late 2002, the Federal government required labels to disclose the presence of trans fats. Listed below are alternatives for popular snacks that are unfortunately high in trans fats. This list, in addition to other acceptable foods, can be found in *Prevention, Healthy Women 2004* by Rodale Inc. Remember that, while these are low in trans fats, total carbohydrates, related to serving size, must be taken into consideration.

Prevention, Healthy Women 2004, chapter 11, "Zero In on the Dangerous Fat," page 78, Rodale, Inc., 2004.

Currently Eating These	Try Eating These
Fleischmann's Original Margarine	Smart Balance Light Buttery Spread
Frito-Lay Sun Chips	Skinny Corn Chips
Kellogg's Low Fat Granola with Raisins	Kashi GoLean Crunch! Cereal
Ore Ida Golden Fries	Ian's Natural foods Sweet Potato fries
Orville Redenbacher's 94% Fat Free Gourmet Popping Corn	Orville Redenbacher's Hot Air Gourmet Popping Corn
Pepperidge Farm Milano Cookies	Barbara's Bakery Double Dutch Chocolate Crisp Cookies
Quaker Fruit & Oatmeal Cereal Bars	Health Valley Strawberry Cobbler Cereal Bars
Stouffer's Lean Cuisine Herb Roasted Chicken	Cascadian Farm Country Herb Chicken with Vegetables & Rice Bowl
Swiss Miss Hot Cocoa Mix, Milk Chocolate	Swiss Miss Hot Cocoa Mix, Diet with calcium
Triscuit Reduced Fat Baked Whole Wheat Crackers	Quilt Whole Wheat Crackers

Other foods that have minimal or no trans fats include:

·   GeniSoy Salted Soy Nuts
·   Mexi-Snax Tortilla Chips
·   Health Valley Fat-Free Apricot Delight
·   Health Valley Original Amaranth Graham Crackers
·   Wasa Healthy Rye Original Crisp Bread
·   Natural Valley Crunchy Granola Bars
·   Pepperidge Farm Natural Whole Grain German Dark Wheat Bread
·   Arnold Natural 100% Whole Wheat Bread
·   General Mills Multi-Bran Chex
·   Kellogg's Complete Wheat Bran Flakes
·   Quaker Toasted Oat Bran Cereal
·   Thomas' Honey Wheat English Muffins
·   Van's All Natural 7 Grain Belgian Waffles
·   Stone Street Bakery Natural Onion-Flavored Cracker Bread
·   Kashi Seven Whole Grains & Sesame TLC
·   Mi-Del Ginger Snaps

Appendix G—Chocolate

Just when you really thought that eating would never be the same again, along comes really great news. CHOCOLATE is good for you. Now, before you start grabbing for the package of Oreo cookies, read the rest of the story. Much like the statement that all fats are not created equal, all chocolates are not created equal. Dark chocolate has been found to be among the highest of the antioxidants (Antioxidant - An agent that inhibits oxidation; any of numerous chemical substances, including certain natural body products and nutrients, which can neutralize the oxidant effect of free radicals and other substances—Stedman's Medical Dictionary). Free radicals have been associated with various types of tissue damage, particularly those involved in atherosclerosis, the aging process, and the development of cancer. Oxidation of LDL cholesterol (the bad cholesterol) appears to be responsible for foam cell formation in the growth of atherosclerotic plaques (clogged arteries). Researchers at the University of California, Davis, discovered that daily consumption of 1 1/3 ounces of *Dove Dark Chocolate* reduced LDL oxidation, boosted antioxidant levels, and increased HDL cholesterol levels. Additionally, they noted reduced blood clotting and stabilization of arterial plaques (making it less likely to become an emboli and travel causing a stroke or heart attack). Remember, it is the percentage of cocoa that provides the antioxidant value—the higher the percentage, the higher the benefit. Joe Vinson, PhD, professor of chemistry at the University of Scranton in Pennsylvania, notes that pure cocoa powder (not sweetened instant hot chocolate) contains the most antioxidants, followed by dark chocolate. Dark chocolate bars generally contain 70% cocoa, and 1 ounce amounts to 11 grams of fat (99 calories). While the dark chocolate, initially, has a somewhat bitter taste, eating it slowly and in combination with fruits and nuts adds to the eating pleasure. Please note that the recommended daily serving is 1.4 ounces, and it must be factored in with total daily calories. When eaten as part of a balanced diet of fruits and vegetables, this food cannot only be a satisfying treat, but also a step toward improved health.

Chocolate Versus Other Antioxidants

Top Antioxidant Foods—ORAC units* per 100 grams

Dark Chocolate	13120
Milk chocolate	6740 **
Prunes	5770
Raisins	2830
Blueberries	2400
Blackberries	2036
Kale	1770
Strawberries	1540
Spinach	1260
Raspberries	1220
Brussel Sprouts	980
Plums	949
Alfalfa Sprouts	930
Broccoli florets	890
Oranges	750
Red Grapes	739
Red Bell Peppers	710
Cherries	670
Onion	450
Corn	400
Eggplant	390

*ORAC (Oxygen Radical Absorbance Capacity) is a measure of the ability of the foods to subdue harmful oxygen free radicals that can damage our bodies. Source: Data from the U.S. Department of Agriculture and the *Journal of the American Chemical Society.*

** There is current research that indicates that eating milk chocolate or eating dark chocolate with dairy products inactivates the antioxidant properties of the chocolate.

Appendix H—Natural Family Planning

The matter of contraception is a personal, and often controversial, matter. Many of the methods available involve introducing estrogen and progestins, at different times, during your monthly cycle. In order to allow the body to stay in hormonal balance, you need to choose a method that does not involve chemically altering your menstrual period. An alternative, the use of condoms, tends to interrupt spontaneity and decrease sensation for the male. Many women complain of irritation or allergic reaction to latex condoms.

Natural family planning (NFP) or fertility awareness has been used successfully for centuries. When practiced correctly, it has a high percentage of effectiveness (reported by various sources ranging from 94.8 to 99.9 percent). For couples planning a pregnancy, understanding the optimal period of fertility will greatly increase the chance for conception. In *Women's Bodies, Women's Wisdom*, authored by Christiane Northrup, M.D., she references a study that reported a 71.4 to 80.9 percent pregnancy rate, within the first cycle, when couples used "fertility-focused intercourse." She notes that the probability of conception in any one cycle, for women with regular menstrual cycles, is 22 to 30 percent. This shows the improved probability for pregnancy, or preventing pregnancy, as a result of knowing the period of increased fertility.

I am going to give a generalized overview of this method, but encourage those interested to utilize the resources at the end of this appendix. Success with fertility awareness requires the education and cooperation of both partners. While many individuals tend to associate this method of contraception with various religions, it is in fact, the only method that works with your body's natural function. By its holistic nature, it tends to draw couples closer and allow both partners to share in the responsibility for conception.

NFP requires that a woman become aware of the subtle aspects of the menstrual cycle that indicate the period of increased fertility. The key is in knowing the time of ovulation. The methods available in determining this include: cervical mucus changes and tracking basal body temperature (BBT).

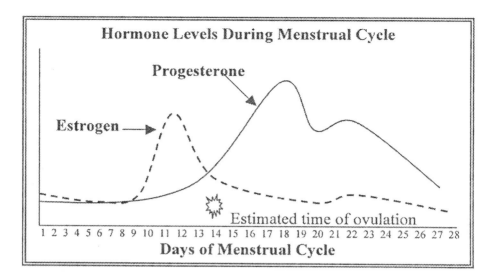

Ovulation is the time of release of an egg (ovum) from the ovary. The second half of your cycle is generally stable at 14 days, and, therefore, in a 28-day cycle, the time of ovulation is estimated to be on day 14. The first half of the cycle is variable and can range from an average of 12 to 17 days. It is this variability that must be tracked in order to accurately predict the period of fertility. As a result of intercourse during the variable period, the chance for pregnancy has been found to increase.

During the latter part of the first half of your cycle, the body begins the process of secreting cervical mucus. At the completion of menstruation, there is no cervical mucus. Christiane Northrup, M.D., refers to this period as "dry" days and indicates that it is generally safe for unprotected sex. At approximately six days prior to ovulation, the presence of E-type mucus (estrogen stimulated mucus) appears. E-type mucus is also referred to as "fertility mucus." It is sticky, clear (it appears to look something like the white of a raw egg), and stretchy when placed between the thumb and forefinger. The purpose of this mucus is to aid in the flow of sperm from the vaginal area, through the cervical opening, and into the uterus. When evaluating for the presence of this type of mucus, look for it around the vaginal opening and vulva, or on the underwear. As soon as you are aware of this type of mucus, you have entered the fertile period. The fertile period extends until the fourth day after peak mucus flow. Peak flow is identified as the last day of flow of the sticky, clear, stretchy type of mucus. Research indicates that ovulation generally occurs two days before or after peak flow.

After the peak flow, one of two changes occurs. The mucus will either change consistency or cease. When the mucus changes, it will become opaque (more yellowish in appearance) and thicker or dense. This type of mucus lacks the elastic, lubricant feature of the E-type mucus. This mucus is referred to as G-type (progesterone stimulated mucus). If mucus discharge stops, you will notice that the vaginal opening again becomes dry. These changes are distinct and indicate that your period will start in 12 to 15 days.

The physiological changes in the first half of the menstrual cycle are related to increasing the chances of pregnancy. The E-type mucus lubricates the vagina and vaginal opening making intercourse easier. Stringy channels, within this type of mucus, help guide sperm through the cervix. Sperm viability, the ability to stay alive, is enhanced by E-type mucus. The thicker, non-sticky G-type mucus actually tends to block the cervix and impede the transfer of sperm between the vagina and uterus.

The second part of Natural Family Planning is determining the time of ovulation, the fertility period, by monitoring basal body temperature (BBT). Progesterone increases as a result of ovulation and is characterized by a temporary rise in basal body temperature. A continued rise in BBT in the second half of the menstrual cycle is indicative of pregnancy.

With this method, you will record your BBT at the beginning of each day throughout your cycle. Day one is the first day of your period (the first day of bleeding). Shake down an oral thermometer before retiring for bed and place it conveniently next to the bed. On awakening, before getting out of bed, place the thermometer snuggly in the armpit for 10 minutes. It is important that the thermometer remain in place for a full 10 minutes. It is also important that the test be completed prior to activity. Record the temperature, numbering the days as noted above (starting with day 1 of your period). The basal body temperature will rise 0.6 to 0.8 degrees F around the time of ovulation and generally remain elevated for 3 consecutive days. The fertile period is considered to be over at the completion of the rise in BBT (that is, when the temperature starts to drop). You should record your daily BBT for a minimum of 3 months. If your cycles are somewhat irregular, you may want to record for 6 months before having unprotected intercourse. In addition to keeping a record of the BBT, record your cervical mucus changes on the same chart. Make note of daily changes with regard to wetness or dryness of the vagina. When mucus is present, note whether it looks like sticky, slippery, egg white (E-type) or thicker and yellowish (G-type). This will give you more information in comparing the changes and increase the reliability of determining the period of fertility.

For couples interested in Natural Family Planning, I encourage you to investigate the following resources:

·   American Academy of Natural Family Planning
www.umkc.edu/sites/hsw/health/birthcontrol/index2.html

·   Family of the Americas
ww.familyplanning.net

·   Couple to Couple League—resource for local teachers and a home study course.
www.ccli.org

·   Billings Ovulation Method
www.billings-centre.ab.ca

·   Natural Family Site
www.bygpub.com/natural/natural-family-planning.htm

·   American Academy of Fertility Care Professionals—resource for finding physicians that support natural family planning.
www.aafc.org

Appendix J—Self Breast Exam (SBE)

Getting to "know" your breasts is one of the best ways to assist your physician in the early detection of breast cancer.

For menstruating women, the best time to do self-breast exam is mid-cycle, when the breast tissue tends to be the least sensitive. It is helpful to know the changes your breasts go through during the monthly cycle, especially if you are prone to fibrocystic breast.

Step 1: Begin by looking at your breasts in the mirror with your shoulders straight and your arms on your hips. Gently press your hands against your hips to tense your chest muscles.

Look for:
· Breasts that are their usual size, shape, and color.
· Breasts that are evenly shaped without visible distortion or swelling.

If you see any of the following changes, bring them to your doctor's attention:
· Dimpling, puckering, or bulging of the skin.
· A nipple that has changed position or an inverted nipple (pushed inward instead of sticking out).
· Redness, soreness, rash, or swelling.

Step 2: Raise your arms above your head, gently pressing your palms together, and look for the same changes outlined in Step 1.

Step 3: While you are at the mirror, gently squeeze each nipple between your finger and thumb and check for nipple discharge.

Step 4: Feel your breasts while you are standing or sitting. Many women find that the easiest way to feel their breasts is when their skin is wet and slippery, so this can be completed while in the shower. Cover your entire breast with soap. Use a firm, smooth touch with the first three fingers of your hand, keeping the fingers flat and together (use the pads of your fingers, not the ends).

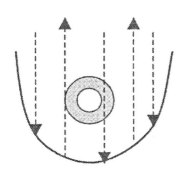 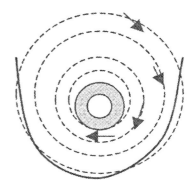

Follow a pattern to be sure that you cover the whole breast. You can begin at the nipple, moving in larger and larger circles until you reach the outer edge of the breast. You can also move your fingers up and down vertically, in rows, as if you were mowing a lawn. Be sure to feel all the breast tissue including the armpit region.

Step 5: Next, feel your breasts while lying down, using your right hand to feel your left breast and then your left hand to feel your right breast. If you have large breasts, it is helpful to raise the arm, on the side of the breast you are examining, above your head. This helps flatten and spread the breast tissue across your chest and ribcage. Cover the entire breast from top to bottom, side to side—from your collarbone to the top of your abdomen, and from your armpit to your cleavage. Begin examining each area with a very soft touch, and then increase pressure so that you can feel the deeper tissue, down to your ribcage.

It is important to feel all the way into the armpit and along the outer portion of the ribcage (directly below the armpit). The area in the upper outer portion of the breast, to the armpit, is a common region to feel a lump. The second most common is at the areola, around the nipple.

In a 10-year study of 266,000 Chinese women, breast self-examination ALONE did not help women live longer. It has been noted that 1 in 4 breast cancers are not picked up on mammogram, but are detected through regular self-examination. The best methods, available now, for detecting breast cancer early are regular BSE, physical examination by a doctor, and mammography—plus use of ultrasound and other tests as needed. Used properly, these tools in combination may increase a woman's chance of surviving breast cancer. In addition, using all of these methods together may help find tumors earlier, when they are smaller, allowing gentler, less invasive and disfiguring treatment options.

Resource: *Journal of the National Cancer Institute, October 2, 2002 and breastcancer.org.*

Appendix J—My Favorite Recipes

Genie Willis' Homemade Pizza

Making Pizza Crusts:

2 cups warm water (heat about 2 minutes in microwave). The temperature of the water should be 105-110 degrees.
3 pkgs. - dry yeast (FLEISCHMANN'S ACTIVE DRY)
1 1/2 T. - honey or sugar

Mix above ingredients together in a large bowl stirring in one direction one hundred times. Proof yeast (this means allow it to rest in bowl for about 10 minutes until you can tell the yeast is active—you will see a bubbling).

Then add:

1 1/2 T. - salt
3 T. - olive oil
3 cups - King Arthur stone-ground, whole-wheat flour
2 cups - King Arthur all-purpose, unbleached flour

Note: You will need about 1 additional cup of unbleached flour for kneading the dough (this can be done on freezer paper, so the dough does not stick).

Mix these ingredients together, then turn out onto a large sheet of floured freezer paper and knead until dough is smooth.

Put kneaded dough into a large greased bowl (cover with plastic wrap) and let rise until doubled in bulk (about 45 minutes).

When the dough has risen, turn out onto floured freezer paper and shape into a long "sausage," then cut into 6 equal pieces.

Preheat oven to 450° with 2 oven racks placed near bottom.

You will need two pizza pans (I recommend the pans with air holes) for baking.

Roll out the first piece of dough into a pizza-sized, round shape; use your hands to make a slightly thicker edge and prick center part of the dough with a fork, to allow air to escape during baking.

Transfer first crust to pizza pan and bake on oven bottom rack.

Roll out the second crust and transfer to second pan.

Switch first crust to upper rack to continue baking. This will allow the top of the first crust to lightly brown. Place the second pizza pan, with the uncooked crust, on the bottom rack.

Roll out third crust, etc.

When barely brown, remove first crust to cooling rack, switch second crust to upper rack, and put third crust in to bake.

Repeat rolling, switching crusts in oven, and baking until all crusts have been baked and cooled.

Freezing Pizza Crusts:

Wrap each crust in freezer paper (reuse the freezer paper from making the crusts) and pack several in large Ziploc freezer bag. Place flat in the freezer for future use.

Making Sauce for a Pizza:

Use a 9"-10" saucepan over medium-to-low heat to reduce the following ingredients almost to paste.

1 can diced tomatoes (14.5 oz.)
2 t. - olive oil
2 garlic cloves (minced)

In lieu of a sauce, you can use tomato slices as the first layer. Cut the tomato across in approximate 1/8-inch slices. Place them on a layer of paper towels, salt, cover with another layer of paper towels, and press lightly to get the moisture out of the tomatoes. Spread them on the precooked crust and then add the other ingredients as directed.

Making the Cheese Topping for a Pizza:

3 oz each Boar's Head Smoked Gruyere & Mozzarella grated
¼ cup fresh Parmesan grated

Making a Pizza:

Preheat oven to 450° with 2 racks in bottom of oven.

To thaw crust, place in oven for about 4-5 minutes, just until it starts to brown.

Using heated sauce (or tomato slices), spread evenly on crust. Add ripe olives, fresh ground pepper. Evenly distribute the cheeses. After baking, top with fresh cut basil leaves.

Bake for about 8-9 minutes.

NOTE: This pizza can be made with all whole-wheat flour or a half and half mix of whole-wheat flour and regular (not white) spelt flour. I do not use any white flour, but if you are not accustomed to working with dough it might be easier to use the whole wheat and white all-purpose flour combination.

Our favorite toppings for pizza are caramelized onions, diced up broccoli, and sliced black olives. Mushrooms would also be good and sliced red, yellow, or green peppers.

Crunchy Granola

Amount	Ingredient
1/2 cup	nonfat dry milk powder -- * see note
1/3 cup	honey
1/3 cup	unsulphured molasses
1/3 cup	apple juice concentrate -- ** see note
2 tablespoons	canola oil
1-tablespoon	vanilla or almond extract
1-tablespoon	cinnamon
1 - 18 oz	package old-fashioned oats
1 cup	almonds cut up, walnuts, or pecans

Add, after baking, while granola cools:
1-cup raisins, dried cherries or cranberries

In a large pot combine the oil, honey, molasses, apple juice concentrate, and nonfat dry milk. Over a low heat stir this until well combined. Remove from heat and stir in the vanilla or almond extract and cinnamon. Pour oats and nuts into the pot and stir well until oats and nuts are evenly coated. Pour the mixture into a large Pyrex pan (I use 11X15) or into 2 smaller pans. Bake at 250 degrees for 1 1/4 to 1 1/2 hours, stirring every 15 minutes to keep top from getting too brown. Add raisins, dried cranberries or cherries when baking is done and oven turned off. Let the granola stay in the oven at least an hour, with the door slightly cracked, until it has completely cooled. This will allow time for the granola to get crisp (sometimes I will let it cool overnight in a closed oven before putting in a large glass container). Store in an airtight container. This does not need to be refrigerated.

*I use the dried soy milk powder (Better Than Milk Dried Soy Light-PLAIN, not flavored!) instead of nonfat dry milk powder. I get this from the health food store. I also get the thin sliced almonds and the dried tart cranberries or cherries out of the health food store bulk bins.

**Apple juice concentrate is found in the freezer section along with other juice concentrates. This granola can be made without the apple juice concentrate (this cuts down on the grams of sugar and carbohydrates).

Chocolate Almond Biscotti

Amount	Ingredient
2 cups	All Purpose Flour (I use white spelt)
1-cup	sugar
1/3 cup	cocoa powder (I use Pernigotti Cocoa from—Williams Sonoma)
1-teaspoon	baking soda
1/4-teaspoon	salt
2	eggs
2	egg whites
3/4-teaspoon	vanilla extract
2/3 cup	toasted almonds (SEE NOTE BELOW)
1/3 cup	Nestles mini chocolate chips

In a stand mixer or in a bowl using a hand mixer, combine the flour, sugar, cocoa powder, baking soda and salt mixing well (or you can sift these to mix well).

Mix together the 2 eggs, 2 more egg whites, and vanilla. Gradually add egg mixture to flour mixture, blending on low. This is a stiff mix at first but mix just until dry ingredients are incorporated. Stir in, by hand, the toasted almonds and the chocolate chips.

Cover dough and place in refrigerator several hours, or overnight, so that the dough will be firmer.

I put freezer paper on my counter and dust it with flour. Divide the dough into two portions and roll into 2 logs ~ 12-14 inches long each. Place on a cookie sheet lined with parchment or grease the cookie sheet. Brush the logs with a beaten egg. Bake at 325 degrees for 30 minutes. Remove from oven and let cool for 15 minutes, then cut with a serrated knife ~3/8 to 1/2 inch slices (if you cut them too thick they will be hard to bite into). Lay the slices on their sides on the baking sheet and return to a 325-degree oven. Bake for about 15 to 20 minutes-do not overcook! Cool and place in an airtight container.

*TOASTED ALMONDS- I buy sliced almonds in the bins at a health food store just for convenience, but the original recipe calls for whole toasted almonds. To toast the almonds: spread a thin layer on a cookie sheet. Put them into a 325-degree oven for 8-10 minutes or until lightly, golden brown. *Pay very close attention* while toasting the almonds. It is easy to *over toast* them!

I get the wonderful cocoa and the Madagascar Bourbon Vanilla from Williams Sonoma.

Salmon Cakes

Amount	Ingredient
2 - 6 OZ	canned pink salmon skinless & boneless
1-teaspoon	Dijon mustard
	lemon juice
	diced onion and diced celery
1/2-cup	fresh toasted breadcrumbs
	salt and pepper
1	whole egg
1	egg white
	fresh parsley

Drain salmon well and flake into small bowl. Add all ingredients except breadcrumbs, mixing well. This can be done in advance and the mixture refrigerated. When ready to cook, add the breadcrumbs, and mix well. Form into 6 patties. In a nonstick pan, heat a small amount of olive or canola oil and place the patties gently into the hot pan. Cook at medium to medium-high heat allowing the first side to brown and then turning to allow the other side to brown (this only takes ~10 minutes for both sides).

BREAD CRUMBS: take a couple slices of bread (I use my homemade spelt bread) and put in blender to make coarse breadcrumbs. To make these crisp I put them on a baking sheet in the oven at 250 degrees until they are golden and crisp. You can make extra and put them in a sealed container in the freezer for future use.

Balsamic Vinegarette Dressing

Amount	Ingredient
1 part	honey or sugar
2 parts	Balsamic Vinegar *see note
	Dijon mustard
	salt and fresh ground pepper
2 parts	canola oil
3 parts	olive oil (Bertolli extra light is good)
small amount	cayenne pepper

For my "1 part" amount, I use a 1/2-cup measuring cup and this makes two bottles of dressing—but you can make a smaller amount. If you want less - just use the same measuring cup size to measure all your parts to this. I put all the ingredients in a blender and pulse it, but you can mix it by hand if you want. If you make it in a blender, do not over blend or it will become overly thick - just pulse it until it is thoroughly mixed.

If you use the 1/2 cup as your "1 part" you will get 4 cups of dressing - for this amount I put in 1 teaspoon salt, and 1 scant tablespoon of Dijon mustard and 1/8- 1/4 teaspoon of cayenne pepper; for a smaller amount of dressing adjust accordingly. Refrigerate after making.

*The Balsamic Vinegar recommended is from Albertson's Modenacett Balsamic Vinegar. It is not expensive for balsamic vinegar and is much better than other brands that I have tried.

$\mathcal{G}lossary$

5

5-HTP
    5-hydroxytryptamine. A precursor to serotonin.

A

acute
    referring to exposure, brief, intense, short-term
ADHD
    a disorder of childhood and adolescence manifested at home, in school, and in
        social situations by developmentally inappropriate degress of inattention,
        impulsiveness, and hyperactivity.
adrenal glands
    one of the endocrine (ductless) glands furnishing internal secretions (epinephrine
        and norepinephrine from the medulla and steroid hormones from the cortex).
Adult Onset Diabetes
    non-insulin-dependent diabetes mellitus. (NIDDM) An often mild form of
        diabetes mellitus of gradual onset, usually in obese individuals over the age
        of 35; absolute plasma insulin levels are normal to high, but relatively low
        in relation to plasma glucose levels; ketoacidosis is rare, but coma can
        occur. Associated with insulin resistance syndrom. Generally controllable
        by dietary means and/or mediation to increase insulin cellular receptors
        sensitivity.
albumin
    a type of simple protein, varieties of which are widely distributed throughout the
        tissues and fluids.
amylase
    one of a group of amylolytic enzymes that cleave starch, glycogen, and related
        glucans.
Anaerobic metabolism
    cellular metabolism that takes place without the presence of oxygen.
androgens
    generic term for an agent, usually a hormone (e.g., androsterone, testosterone),
        that stimulates activity of the accessory male sex organs, encourages
        development of male sex characteristics.

angiogenesis
> the development of new blood vessels needed to feed the growth of cancer cells.

B

benign
> denoting the mild or uncomplicated character of an illness or the nonmalignant character of a cancer.

biotransformation
> the process of metabolizing and changing the form of a toxin in order to store or excrete it.

Black Cohosh
> *cimicifuga racemosa*. A herb used for the treatment of menopausal symptoms, especially hot flashes. Should not be used by patients taking anti-hypertensive medication. Should be used for no more that six to twelve months.

C

calories
> a unit of heat content or energy. The amount of heat necessary to raise one gram of water from 14.5-15.5 degrees Centigrade. A measure utilized to calculate food consumption versus body energy expenditure.

carpal tunnel syndrome
> compression of the median nerve as it courses under the ligaments of the wrist. Symptoms include numbness and tingling, pain, and muscle wasting in the hand and fingers (especially the middle finger).

cell receptors
> a structural protein molecule on the cell surface or within the cytoplasm that binds to a specific factor, such as a drug, homrmone, antigen, or neurotransmitter. Can be though of as a lock and key type connection.

cellulose
> forms the basis of vegetable and wood fiber and is the most abundant organic compound.

cholesterol
> the most abundant steroid in animal tissues, especially in bile and gallstones, and present in food, especially food rich in animal fats.

chronic
> referring to exposure, prolonged or long-term.

chymotrypsin
> Chymotrypsin A or B

citric acid
> The acid of citrus fruits, widely distributed in nature and a key intermediate in intermediary metabolism.

clinical
> Denoting the symptoms and course of a disease, as distinguished from the laboratory findings of anatomical changes.

COPD
> Abbreviation for chronic obstructive pulmonary disease.

cruciferous vegetables
> A group of vegetables that includes: brocolli, cabbage, cauliflower, kale, turnip greens, collard greens, brussel sprouts, and mustard greens. Contains indole-3-carbinol, an anti-inflammatory.

D

degenerative disease
> Also known as osteoarthritis. Arthritis characterized by erosion of articular cartilage, either primary or secondary to trauma or other conditions, which becomes soft, frayed, and thinned. Pain and loss of function result.

DEXA scan
> A radiographic procedure for determining the mineralization, density, of bone. Associated with the evaluation of osteoporosis.

dextrose
> A dextrorotatory monosaccharide (hexose) found in the free state in fruits and other parts of plants.

DHEA
> Abbreviation for dehydroepiandrosterone. One of the steroid sex hormones.

disaccharides
> A condensation product of two monosaccharides by elimination of water (usually between an alcoholic OH and a hemiacetal OH).

down-regulate
> The ability for a hormone or chemical to decrease the activity of a metabolic function.

E

endocrine disruption
> Chemicals that mimic estrogen activity and cause abnormal endocrine activity.

ERT
> Abbreviation for estrogen replacement therapy.

Estrogen dominance
> A relative increase of estrogen and estrogen-like metabolic activity to the amount of progesterone activity.

estrogens
> Generic term for any substance, natural or synthetic, that exerts biologic effects characteristic of estrogenic hormones such as 17*-estradiol. Estrogens are formed by the ovary, placenta, testes, and possibly the adrenal cortex, as well as by certain plants.

F

fibromyalgia
> A syndrome of chronic pain of musculoskeletal origin but uncertain cause. The American College of Rheumatology has established diagnostic criteria that include pain on both sides of the body, both above and below the waist, as well as in an axial distribution (cervical, thoracic, or lumbar spine or anterior chest).

Free calcium
> The amount of blood calcium above an optimal level (noted as 2.5 times blood phosphorus).

fructose
> Fruit sugar. Does not cause the initial rise in insulin like glucose when ingested. Is metabolized in the liver to glucose

functional medicine
> A holistic approach to healthcare, including integrating aspects of allopathic and structural medicine.

functional thoracic outlet syndrome (TOS)
> A condition resulting from compression of the brachial plexus (nerves from the neck to arms) at the region above the collar bone. Symptoms can include numbness & tingling in the arm and hand, especially on the little finger side.

G

GERD
> Abbreviation for gastrointestinal esophageal reflux disease.

GI
> Gastrointestinal. Having to do with the digestive tract, including the esophagus to the rectum.

GLA
> Abbreviation for gamma linolenic acid, an omega-6 essential fatty acid (EFA).

glucagon
> A form of sugar storage in the liver.

glycemic index
> A ranking of the rise in serum glucose from various foodstuffs.

glycemic load
> The glycemic index multiplied by a carbohydrates density.

glycogen
> the principal carbohydrate reserve, it is readily converted into glucose.

GMP
> Abbreviation for Good Manufacturing Practices.

H

HIPPA
   Health Insurance Portability and Accountability Act (Federal
      Government—1996).
HRT
   Abbrviation for hormone replacement therapy; contains both estrogen and
      progesterone.
hyperglycemia
   Elevated blood sugar.
hypertension
   High blood pressure.
hypoglycemia
   Low blood sugar.
hypothalamus
   A structure of the brain responsible for directing hormonal activity. The
      hypothalamus is prominently involved in the functions of the autonomic
      (visceral motor) nervous system and, through its vascular link with the
      anterior lobe of the hypophysis, in endocrine mechanisms.

I

innervation
   The supply of nerve fibers functionally connected with a part.
insoluble fiber
   Fiberous products that are incapable of dissolving in the intestine. Aids bowel
      movement by attracting water to the fecal matter.
insulin resistance syndrome
   see Metabolic Syndrome.
Integrative Medicine
   see Functional Medicine.
ischemic heart disease
   Inadequate circulation of blood to the heart muscle, usually as a result of
      coronary artery disease.

J

joints
   In anatomy, the place of union, usually more or less movable, between two or
      more bones

L

lactic acid
A normal intermediate in the fermentation of sugar. In pure form, a syrupy, odorless, and colorless liquid obtained by the action of the lactic acid bacillus on milk or milk sugar.

lecithin
Phospholipids that are found in nervous tissue, especially in the myelin sheaths, in egg yolk, and as essential constituents of animal and vegetable cells.

ligaments
A band or sheet of fibrous tissue connecting two or more bones, cartilages, or other structures, or serving as support for fasciae or muscles.

lipid
Associated with fat and cholesterol.

M

macromanage
The use of management techniques that consider the whole or total.

malic acid
An acid found in apples and various other tart fruits.

maltose
Malt sugar. A disaccharide formed in the breakdown of starch.

melatonin
N -Acetyl-5-methoxytryptamine.

Metabolic Syndrome
Also known as Syndrome X. A condition marked by elevated blood glucose and insulin—a precursor to Adult Onset Diabetes (Type II).

mitochondria
An organelle in the cellular cytoplasm, referred to as cellular factories or furnaces

monosaccharides
A carbohydrate that cannot form any simpler sugar by simple hydrolysis.

mucosa
A mucous tissue lining various tubular structures, consisting of epithelium, lamina, propria, and, in the digestive tract, a layer of smooth muscle.

muscles
One of the contractile tissues of the body by which movements of the various organs and parts are effected.

N

NSAID
The abbreviation for non steroidal anti-inflammatory drug. Non prescription examples include: Aleve, Advil, Nuprin, and generic ibuprofen. Prescription examples include: Celebrex, Vioxx, and Naprosyn.

O

occlusion
The act of closing or the state of being closed.
Omega-3 fatty acids
A polyunsaturated essential fatty acid, characterized by it's bonding structure.

osteoporosis
Reduction in the quantity of bone or atrophy of skeletal tissue.

P

pancreatin
A mixture of the enzymes from the pancreas of the ox or hog, used internally as
a digestive, and also as a peptonizing agent in preparing predigested foods.
papain
A proteolytic enzyme found in papaya used as a protein digestant, meat
tenderizer, and to prevent adhesions.
pepsin
Pepsin A is the principal digestive enzyme of gastric juice.
pH
The measure of the hydrogen ion concentration of a substance. A pH of 7 denotes
neutral. A pH less than 7 is noted as acidic, above 7 as basic or alkaline.
phagocyte
A cell possessing the property of ingesting bacteria, foreign particles, and other
cells.
physiological
Denoting the various vital bodily functions.
phytoestrogen
Plant based substances that have an estrogenic affect on cellular receptors. Plant
products that behave biologically similar to natural estrogen.
pituitary gland
A small gland suspended from the hypothalamus (on the bottom side of the brain)
responsible for secretion of somatotropins, prolactin, thyroid-stimulating
hormone, gonadotropins, adrenal corticotropin, and other related peptides.
preferentially
When a hormone or chemical will bind at a cellular receptor site first, or easier
than another hormone.
progesterone
An antiestrogenic steroid, believed to be the active principle of the corpus
luteum, isolated from the corpus luteum and placenta. Generic term for any
substance, natural or synthetic, that effects some or all of the biologic
changes produced by progesterone. Sometimes used incorrectly for
progestin, which is a synthetic form of progesterone.

Progestin
> A synthetic chemical that simulates the activity of progesterone. Not to be confused with the body's natural progesterone or bioidentically produced progesterone.

Prognosis
> A forecast of the probable course and/or outcome of a disease.

Proteins
> The primary structural material, consisting of strings of amino acids. Makes up approximately 75% of cell matter. Involved in the make-up of hormones, enzymes, immulogical factors, etc.

proteolytic enzyme
> Digestive protein that assists in the breakdown or change of dietary protein.

R

receptor site
> The point of attachment for viruses, hormones, or other activators to cell membranes

---

S

satiety
> The state produced by fulfillment of a specific need, such as hunger or thirst.

serotonin
> A neurotransmitter /hormone. It acts as a vasoconstrictor, liberated by blood platelets, that inhibits gastric secretion and stimulates smooth muscle.

soluble fiber
> Fiber that is capable of dissolving. In the intestines this form of fiber turns to a gel-like substance that assists in slowing digestion

St Johns Wort
> A herb that is associated with treatment of mild to moderate depressive states.

statin
> A form of medication used for management of hyperlipidemia, elevated cholesterol.

subclinical
> Denoting the presence of a disease without manifest symptoms.

sucrose
> A nonreducing disaccharide made up of D-glucose and D-fructose obtained from sugar cane, from several species of sorghum, and from the sugar beets

Syndrome X
> See Metabolic Syndrome

T

tendons
> A nondistensible fibrous cord or band of variable length that is the part of the muscle that connects the fleshy (contractile) part of muscle with its bony attachment.

trypsin
> A proteolytic enzyme formed in the small intestine from trypsinogen by the action of enteropeptidase

---

U

up-regulate
> The ability for a hormone or chemical to increase the activity of a metabolic function.

USP
> Abbreviation for United States Pharmacopeia.

V

Vitex
> *vitex agnus castus*, also known as Chaste Tree. A herb thought to enhance the natural production of progesterone and lutenizing hormone in the second half of the menstrual cycle. Should not be used during pregnancy or lactation   96

X

xenobiotics
> See xenoestrogens

xenoestrogens
> By-products of industrial and chemical processing that tend to mimic the activity of estrogen and other hormones when attached to a cellular receptor.

References

Texts:

"Adrenocortex Stress Profile." *Functional Assessment Resource Manual.* North Carolina: GSDL, Winter 2002.

Atkins, R. *Atkins for Life.* USA: St. Martin's Press, 2003.

Agatston, Arthur. *The South Beach Diet.* USA: St. Matins Press, 2003.

Barnes, B and Galton, L. *Hypothyroidism, the Unsuspected Illness.* New York: Harper & Row, 1976.

"Bone Resorption Assessment." *Functional Assessment Resource Manual.* North Carolina: GSDL Winter 2002.

Brownstein, D. *The Miracle of Natural Hormones.* 2003. Michigan: Medical Alternatives Press, 1998.

"Female Hormone Profile." *Functional Assessment Resource Manual.* North Carolina: GSDL Winter 2002.

Gray, K. *Eat and Be Well.* USA: Krystal Gray, 2002.

Guyton, A and Hall, J. *Textbook of Medical Physiology.* 2000. Philadelphia: W B Saunders. 1956.

"Healthy Women 2004." *Prevention.* Emmaus, PA: Rodale Inc, 2004.

Lee, J, Hopkins, V., and Hanley, J. *What Your Doctor May Not Tell You About Menopause.* USA: Time Warner, 1996.

Lee, John, et al. *What Your Doctor May Not Tell You About Premenopause.* USA: Time Warner, 1999.

Lee, J, Hopkins, V, and Zava, D. *What Your Doctor May Not Tell You About Breast Cancer*. USA: Time Warner, 2002.

Love, S and Lindsey, K. *Dr. Susan Love's Menopause and Hormone Book*. 2003. New York: Three Rivers Press, 1997.

"Menopause Profile." *Functional Assessment Resource Manual*. North Carolina: GSDL Winter 2002.

Northrup, C. *Women's Bodies, Women's Wisdom*. 1998. New York: Bantam Books, 1994.

Northrup, C. *The Wisdom of Menopause*. 2003. New York: Bantam Books, 2001.

Pearson, C et al. *The Truth About Hormone Replacement Therapy*. USA: Prima Publishing, 2002.

Pert, C. *Molecules of Emotion*. New York: Scribner, 1997.

Rakowski, R. *Understanding the Clinical Applications of Improved Metabolic Biotransformation*. Washington, Metagenics Educational Programs, 2003.

Regelson, W and Colman, C. *The Super Hormone Promise*. New York: Simon and Schuster, 1996.

Schwartz, E. *The Hormone Solution*. USA: Time Warner, 2002.

Schwarzbein, D. and Deville, N. *The Schwarzbein Principle*. Deerfield Beach: Health Communications, 1999.

Schwarzbein, Diane and Brown, M. *The Schwarzbein Principle II—The Transition*. Deerfield Beach: Health Communications, 2002.

Seaman, B. *The Greatest Experiment Ever Performed*. USA: Hyperion Books, 2003.

Sears, Barry. *The Omega Rx Zone*. New York: HarperCollins Books, 2002.

Steward, H et al. *Sugar Buster! Cut Sugar to Trim Fat.* 1998. USA: Ballantine Publishing, 1995.

"Zero In on the Dangerous Fat." *Prevention, Healthy Women 2004.* USA: Rodale, 2004:78.

Articles:

"A Woman's Heart." BioAging Inc. *np.*

"An Overview of Syndrome X." Florida: Professional Co-op Services, 2002.

"Beauty: Inside Info." Health June 2004: 42.

"Beware: Breast implants can Fool mammograms." Health June 2004: 55.

Chen, R and Tunstall-Pedoe, H. "Coronary Heart Disease in Relation to Passive Smoking - Scottish Monica Study." (Cardiovascular Epidemiology Unit, Ninewells Hospital and Medical School, Dundee, UK), *Abstracts of the Society for Epidemiologic Research*, June 2003.

Condor, B. "Women With Chest Pain Spoke Up and Lived." *Tallahassee Democrat* February 10, 2003.

Dranov, P. "Can We End Heart Disease for Good?" *Ladies Home Journal* Apr 2004: 176-186.

Guilliams, T. "Female Cycle Difficulties." *The Standard* Vol. 4, No. 2, 2001.

Guilliams, T. "Menopause - A Natural Transition." *The Standard* Vol. 4, No.1, 2001.

Gorman, C. "The No 1 Killer of Women." *Time* April 28, 2003.

Gorman, C and Park. A. "The Fires Within." *Time* Feb 23, 2004: 39-46.

Haney, D. "Study: Exercise Improves Cancer Survival." *Tallahassee Democrat* March 31, 2004.

"Hidden Sugars Lie in Wait for Children." *Atlanta-Journal Constitution Online* April 1, 2004.

Jones, B et al. "Obesity and Survival in a Cohort of African American and White Women with Breast Cancer." (Yale University School of Medicine, New Haven, CT). *Abstracts of the Society for Epidemiologic Research*, June 2003.

Kruger, J, et al. "Are Adults Achieving the Recommended Physical Activity Level for Losing Weight?" (Centers for Disease Control and Prevention, Atlanta, GA). *Abstracts of the Society for Epidemiologic Research*, June 2003.

Leaf. C. "Why We're Losing the War on Cancer." *Fortune* Vol 149, No 6: 77-97.

McElroy, J, et al. "Exposure to Plasticizers and Breast Cancer Risk." (University of Wisconsin, Madison, WI). *Abstracts of the Society for Epidemiologic Research*, June 2003.

"Mercury in Seafood: How Much is Safe?" *Low Carb Living*. Vol. 1, No 2: 29.

Pathak, D, et al. "Reduced Cabbage/Sauerkraut is Associated with Increased Breast Cancer." (Michigan State University, Lansing, MI). *Abstracts of the Society for Epidemiologic Research*, June 2003.

Paturel, A. "How to Read a Food Label." *Shape* June 2004: 188-191.

"Self Breast Examination." *Journal of the National Cancer Institute*. October 2, 2002.

"Self Breast Examination." www.breastcancer.org.

"10 Harmful Ingredients In Personal Care Products." www.bestchoice.itgo.com.

Tallmadge, K. "Carb Control [the smart way]" *Shape* June 2004: 219-224.

"Ten Synthetic Cosmetic Ingredients to Avoid." *Organic Consumers Association* www.organicconsumers.org.

Title Nine Sports Catalogue, title9sports.com. Summer 2004.

Uhlenhuth, K. "Betcha Can't Eat Just One." *Tallahassee Democrat* February 10, 2003.

United States. Federal Drug Administration. FDA Consumer—Consumer Ingredients. *Cosmetic Ingredients: Understanding the Puffery*. Revised February 1995.

United States. Federal Drug Administration. FDA Consumer—Cosmetic Safety. *Cosmetic Safety: More Complex Than at First Blush*. Revised May 1995.

United States. National Institutes of Health. *Clinical Guidelines on the Identification, Evaluation, and Treatment of Overweight and Obesity in Adults*, Bethesda, MD, 1998.

Van Oyen, H, et al. "Young Adult Smokers Are Less Likely to Have Healthy Nutritional Habits." (Scientific Institute of Public Health, Brussels, Belgium). *Abstracts of the Society for Epidemiologic Research*, June 2003.

Vasan, R, et al. "Residual Lifetime Risk for Developing Hypertension in Middle-aged Men and Women." (The Framingham Heart Study.) *JAMA* 287(8) (2002).

Weuve, J., Kang, JH, and Grodstein, F. "Physical activity and Cognitive Function." (Harvard Medical School, Boston, MA). *Abstracts of the Society for Epidemiologic Research* June 2003.

"Which Vitamins Prevent Chronic Disease?" *JAMA* 287(23) 2002.

Yee, D (AP). "Carbs Culprit in Women's Weight Gain." *Tallahassee Democrat* February 6, 2004.

Yee, D (AP). "Weight, Breast Cancer Tied Weight Gain." *Denver Post* Feb 26, 2004.

Printed in the United States
28105LVS00005B/209